OXFORD MEDICAL PUBLICATIONS

BORN TOO EARLY

BORN TOO EARLY

Special care
for your
preterm baby

Margaret Redshaw
Research Psychologist,
formerly of the Perinatal Research Unit,
St Mary's Hospital,
London

Rodney Rivers
Reader in Paediatrics,
St Mary's Hospital Medical School,
London

Deborah Rosenblatt
Senior Research Psychologist,
Sam Segal Perinatal
St Mary's Hospital Medical School,
London

Oxford   New York   Toronto
OXFORD UNIVERSITY PRESS
1985

Oxford University Press, Walton Street, Oxford OX2 6DP
London New York Toronto
Delhi Bombay Calcutta Madras Karachi
Kuala Lumpur Singapore Hong Kong Tokyo
Nairobi Dar es Salaam Cape Town
Melbourne Auckland
and associated companies in
Beirut Berlin Ibadan Mexico City Nicosia

Oxford is a trade mark of Oxford University Press

British Library Cataloguing in Publication Data

Redshaw, Margaret
Born too early.
1. Infants (Premature)
I. Title   II. Rivers, Rodney
III. Rosenblatt, Deborah
618.92'011   RJ250
ISBN 0-19-261542-4
ISBN 0-19-261427-4 (pbk.)

Library of Congress Cataloging in Publication Data

Redshaw, Margaret
Born too early.
(Oxford medical publications)
Includes bibliographies and index.
1. Infants (Premature)—Care and hygiene.
I. Rivers, Rodney. II. Rosenblatt, Deborah.
III. Title. IV. Series [DNLM: 1. Infant Care.
2. Infant, Premature. WS 410 R321b]
RJ250.R43 1984   618.92'011   84-14732
ISBN 0-19-261542-4
ISBN 0-19-261427-4 (pbk.)

Printed and bound in Great Britain by
Butler & Tanner Ltd.
Frome and London

Foreword

George Pinker, CVO, FRCS, FRCOG
Consultant Obstetrician and Gynaecologist
St. Mary's Hospital, London

The team of nurses, doctors, psychologists, and social workers who have staffed the intensive and special care baby unit at St. Mary's Hospital have revolutionized the care available to preterm babies; they have given them not only the chance of life but of living normally, and this work is mirrored in many other such units all over the Western World.

These dedicated workers perhaps know better than anyone the stresses and strains which the parents are exposed to when their baby is born too early. In this book the authors have concisely yet compassionately looked at the causes, the delivery, and the special problems which result from the birth of a preterm baby.

They outline the facilities that are available, the way in which decisions are taken at the time of the birth and afterwards, and the way in which the parents and family can become the most important part of the team caring for the baby after its birth. They have sensed the problems which face the parents and the immediate family and have given clear answers to the questions which will occur to them and explanations of the various procedures and experiences which are likely to happen.

I believe that this book will do a great deal to help those who initially are alarmed at the turn of events and need every help to be able to get their problems into perspective. The text is clear, professionally educative, and reassuring. I feel sure that it will help parents who find themselves in the circumstances of having a preterm baby to face the problems which lie ahead with much greater calm and understanding.

Acknowledgements

Without exposure to the infectious optimism and endeavours in the field of neonatal medicine arising in the 1960s, this book might never have been written. Early influences created an awareness of the importance of an interdisciplinary approach to the problems of preterm babies and their families. Our questioning, humanistic mentors of that time included Professors Leonard Strang and Osmund Reynolds, Drs Robert Boyd and Jonathan Shaw, Anthea Blake, Lily Dubowitz, Joanna Hawthorne-Amick, and Dianne Melvin. They made lasting impressions on us and, by their example, are to be credited with having stimulated us during formative years.

We are now most fortunate in having Professors Richard Beard, Tom Oppé, and Brian Foss as departmental heads; their wisdom and insight in recognizing the importance of marrying the disciplines of obstetrics, paediatrics, and psychology and in stimulating activity in perinatal investigation and care ensures that the emotional needs of families with a high risk pregnancy receive as much attention as do their physical problems.

We are immensely appreciative of our families for their tolerance of our engrossment—the late nights and weekend working. We would also like to thank the many authors and teachers whose work we have drawn on and our friends who have contributed their ideas, comments, and criticisms of the text, particularly Linda Reid, Wendy Cartwright, Anne Seymour, Didi Macedo, Phil Steer, Joan Greenwood, Sharon Cavanagh, and Tom Lissauer. We cannot name all the doctors and nurses with whom we have been privileged to work and who have devoted themselves to the high standards of perinatal care and the creation of a caring environment which we have tried to reflect in the book; however Nellie Wood has been foremost amongst our neonatal unit sisters in facilitating the integration of clinical care and research there.

We are indebted to Sue Madge for her limitless tolerance of our manuscript alterations and for her dedicated typing of them. We gratefully acknowledge the expertise of our photographic department, and in particular Ann Marie; they have been superb in the processing and reproduction of the photographs. Charts depicting weight and head circumferences have been adapted from the chart prepared by Drs D. Gairdner and J. Pearson, published by Castlemead Publications, Hertford. The chart of biparietal diameters was adapted from Campbell.

Our greatest debt of gratitude is to the many families over the years who have entrusted their newborns to our care. They accepted our frequent observation and testing of their babies and the discussion of their problems and feelings, all while trying to get on with the day-to-day demands of parenting a preterm baby. Many of them have been most generous in allowing us to use treasured photographs, to quote their personal views and experiences, and, in the instance of Ann Lawrence, to reproduce her poem.

Note

The authors and publisher of this book have, as far as is possible, taken care to ensure that descriptions of practice and recommendations regarding care of preterm babies are correct and compatible with current standards of treatment. Medical science is constantly advancing and as new information becomes available some of these practices will change.

An individual's care is the responsibility of the medical staff concerned and they are the best source of information about your own baby's condition. The explanations and suggestions offered do not replace the need for obtaining professional health advice for your infant.

Contents

Introduction

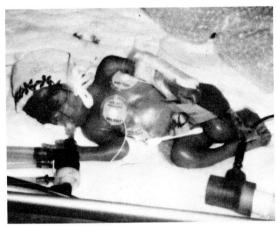

Simone

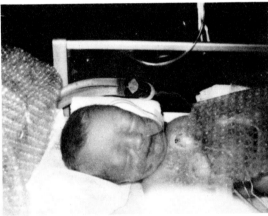

Oliver

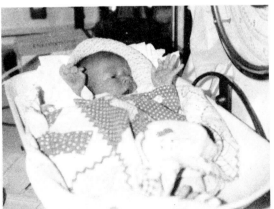

Kim

Simone arrived 15 weeks ahead of schedule, weighing in at only 820 g (1 lb 13 oz). Because of her mother's two 'bleeds' during the preceding week and her very early gestation of 25 weeks the obstetricians delivered her by Caesarean section. Two doses of a steroid (betamethasone) given to her mother in the 48 hours before delivery probably helped her lungs mature a little before birth. None the less she spent her first 56 days on a ventilator in the intensive care unit and then another 20 days in a headbox receiving oxygen until she was finally breathing room air on her own at 11 weeks of age. She developed a loud heart murmur and required medication to close her patent ductus arteriosus. Altogether she needed 21 blood transfusions during her stay. Simone received most of her nutritional needs intravenously for seven weeks, but also had expressed breast milk and formula feeds by tube. When she was able to finish all her bottles, she finally went home to her parents and sisters after 15 weeks in hospital, just about the day that she was expected to be born.

Oliver was born by emergency Caesarean section because of the sudden, life-threatening, partial separation of his placenta. At birth he seemed well and was a good weight—2.0 kg (4 lb 6 oz)—for his gestation of 33 weeks. Possibly as a result of sustaining blood loss during the placental separation, he was found to have a low blood pressure and he developed progressive breathing difficulties due to the immaturity of his lungs. He needed breathing support from a ventilator and 100 per cent oxygen to maintain adequate oxygenation of his blood. However by 11 days he was breathing air by himself.

At two weeks, when all seemed to be going well, his head was noted to be increasing rapidly in size. Ultrasound examination confirmed that there was raised pressure in the fluid-filled chambers of his brain and repeated removal of fluid by lumbar puncture was required in order to reduce the pressure. Oliver's 'lumbar taps' were eventually discontinued as the condition stabilized by 15 weeks of age, although his parents had been able to take him home six weeks before.

By the time Kim arrived at 36 weeks' gestation, weighing 2.860 kg (6 lb 5 oz), the obstetric and paediatric staff were old friends of the family. Her father was a porter at the hospital and her two-year-old sister, Gemma, had herself been admitted to the neonatal unit as she had been born eight weeks early; this time her mother had spent the last 12 weeks of her 'high-risk' pregnancy in the antenatal ward three doors down from the intensive care nursery.

Although her mother's previous obstetric experience together with a series of tests during the pregnancy had indicated that Kim was likely to be small for her gestational age, no-one anticipated any particular problems; the breathing difficulties associated with being born early are less common by 36 weeks' gestation. To everyone's surprise she was a bumper size, but she developed mild respiratory distress syndrome. She required breathing support for a few days, followed by three days in a headbox receiving oxygen before she was finally breathing room air at one week of age.

She was started on tube feeds but soon mastered the art of sucking from a bottle. Even the two weeks she remained in the neonatal unit seemed endless to her parents, and brought back memories of their older daughter's many problems two years before.

Despite their very different gestations, birthweights, and obstetric and neonatal experiences, all these babies shared a common beginning to their lives—they were preterm. Born too early to survive without intensive medical technology, they relied on a dedicated team of nurses and doctors to monitor their temperature, breathing, and nutritional needs, and to diagnose problems and treat them appropriately.

For their parents the usual anticipated normal delivery and short hospital stay were suddenly replaced by a stressful birth followed by weeks of anxiety and distress. Only slowly could they come to assume their full-time role as parents and feel the satisfaction of meeting their baby's every need.

1

What is a
preterm baby?

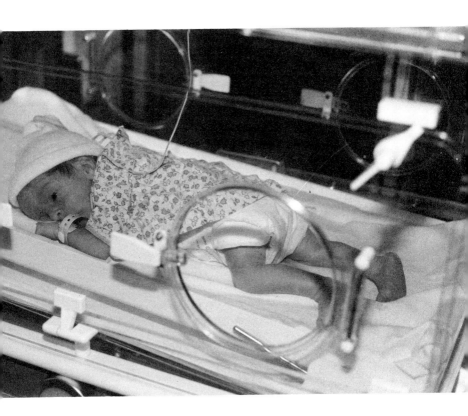

M any people are uncertain about the meaning of the word 'preterm'. Preterm, or premature babies as they used to be called, are those who have been born too soon. They are immature and their problems are mainly due to the fact that some body systems are not ready to take on the various functions and activities necessary for healthy survival after birth. Babies born 'at term' have reached an optimal stage of development and maturity, and when given warmth, food, affection, and appropriate care, are capable of 'independent' survival. Babies who are born *before the 37th week* of pregnancy are considered preterm.

Not all babies who have a low weight at birth are actually preterm. Some are babies who have reached a level of maturity appropriate for their term gestation (more than 37 weeks) but have failed to put on weight normally. These babies are referred to as small for gestational age (SGA). Their low weight can be the result of various growth-restricting influences acting at different phases of intra-uterine development. Such infants, though born at the right time, are therefore small in comparison with other term newborns. In the past all small babies were thought of as 'premature'. The recognition of the distinction between preterm and small for gestational age babies has enabled paediatricians to provide appropriate supportive care for the very differing requirements of each group. The terms applied to the baby at various stages of development during pregnancy are indicated in Table 1.1.

Gestational age

This is defined as the number of completed weeks of pregnancy from the last menstrual period. The gestational age is calculated from data provided by the mother concerning the date of her last menstrual period and the length and regularity of her cycle. An ultrasound scan of the fetus prior to 18 weeks of age can provide confirmation of the gestational age and of the calculated date of delivery.

Use of ultrasound

Ultrasound techniques are not only becoming more widely available but also more sophisticated, and now provide images of excellent quality. During a scan, the fetus is exposed to very brief

Table 1.1

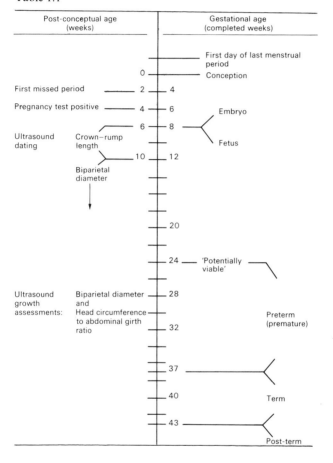

pulses of high frequency sound-waves. Most of the scanning time is actually taken up with the collection of the echoes (reflections) of the sound-waves as they return to the scan head. Imagine waves generated by dropping a pebble into still water in a bath tub, spreading out, striking the side, and 'bouncing' back. Since body tissues of differing composition give rise to echoes of varying intensity when exposed to these sound-waves, a 'picture' can be constructed electronically from the strength and pattern of the echoes received. Measurements can then be made from the screened image, provided of course that the fetus remains in a suitable position for long enough.

An ultrasound scan carried out before the 18th week of pregnancy is an important way of confirming the gestational age of a fetus, for up to this time there is little variation between individuals of the same age in some of the body measurements that can be made. Differences in size between babies become more marked as pregnancy progresses so that later on such measurements are less useful as a means of deciding the age of a particular fetus. Early measurements are most likely to be taken from the crown of the head to the rump ('crown–rump' length, CRL). By 16 weeks, the width of the fetal head—the so-called 'biparietal diameter' (BPD)—is a more accurate measurement. The progressive increase in biparietal diameter during pregnancy is normally a reflection of the rate of the baby's brain growth. It can be a useful indicator of a baby's well-being.

From repeated measurements made on many babies normal rates of increase in head growth have been reported; deviations from the norm can therefore be detected. In the last weeks of pregnancy, ultrasound scans may be used to make measurements of the baby's abdominal (tummy) girth. At this stage of pregnancy energy reserves are accumulating in the baby's liver. If the level of nutrition is less than optimal the liver size, and thus the size of the fetus's abdomen, will not increase at the normal rate. Since individual babies vary in size there are problems in interpreting the significance of a single measurement, and so a ratio is produced which combines the head circumference and abdomen measurements. Using this ratio it is possible to pick out some of those babies whose level of nutrition may be inadequate, because of an unfavourable intra-uterine environment, since in these the rate of abdominal growth lags behind that of head growth.

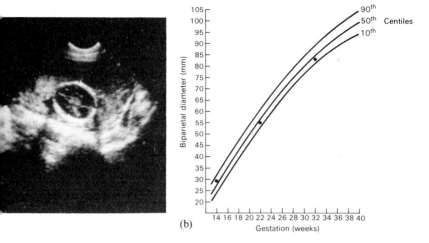

(a) The ultrasound picture of the fetus shows the parietal contours of the head. The greatest distance between the parietal contours is taken as the biparietal diameter.

(b) The measurement is plotted on a chart according to the gestation at the time of scanning; sequential measurements give an indication of brain growth. Early u/s ruled out the presence of twins in this 'large-for-dates' pregnancy and the serial scans indicate that the head is growing close to the 50th centile.

Growth charts

All measurements of growth whether of length, weight, abdominal girth, biparietal diameter, or head circumference, can be related to the range of values obtained from a 'normal' population. Unfortunately, few published charts take into account the effects of influences such as the number of completed previous pregnancies, or a mother's stature, on the dimensions of the baby. Some babies may be small because their mothers are. None the less these measurements can provide a useful reference for detecting significant deviations from the normal pattern of growth, especially when taken at intervals over the pregnancy.

By taking as many as 1000 newborns at a given gestation, charts have been constructed which indicate the limits that encompass the closest 80 per cent of the measurements, and thus the levels at which 10 per cent of the babies would be more and 10 per cent less, than the other 80 per cent of babies for the particular measurement under consideration. For weight, we can therefore define babies who are large for their gestational age (LGA) as being above the

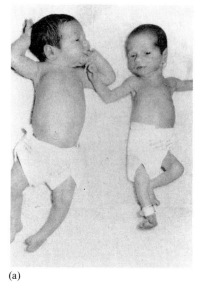

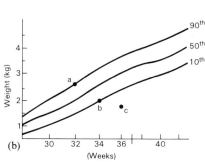

(a)   (b)

(a) One of these 36-week gestation twins is small for her gestational age (SGA); her sister is of appropriate size.

(b) Weight chart with the birth weights of three preterm babies plotted.
    (a) This baby at 32 weeks is heavier than 90 per cent of babies born at that gestation.
    (b) Only 10 babies weigh less than this one at 34 weeks gestation and he is 'borderline' SGA.
    (c) This baby is preterm and very growth retarded; there are less than 3 out of every 100 babies at 36 weeks who would weigh as little as this at birth.

90th centile, and those who are small for their gestational age (SGA) as being below the 10th centile lines. Babies whose weights are anywhere between these lines, are regarded as 'normal', but they *may* be normal even when outside these limits. However, it is more likely for a baby who has experienced a stressful intra-uterine environment to be found in the extreme centiles.

Babies below the 10th centile line for weight at a given gestation can be described as being small for gestational age (SGA), or small for dates (SFD). Sometimes these descriptions are reserved for the 3 per cent of babies below the 3rd centile line. There is no universal agreement for the designation 'small for gestational age'.

The importance of identifying babies who are small for gestational age derives from observations that some of these babies need extra nutrients in the first few days of life. This is because they lack the necessary energy stores to maintain an adequate sugar level in the bloodstream, and they are usually given glucose (dextrose) solutions in addition to their 'feeds'.

Babies who are born prematurely can *also* be small for their gestational age. Indeed, obstetricians may decide that it is better to deliver a baby early who is not growing well in the uterus. It can be safer to adopt this course of action when there is intra-uterine growth retardation (IUGR) than to allow the pregnancy to continue. Allowing continuation of the pregnancy may sometimes further reduce the baby's ability to tolerate the stress of labour, and might even result in the birth of a 'stillborn' infant.

How frequently does preterm birth occur?

About seven out of every 100 babies are born before completion of the 37th week of gestation. This means that in the United Kingdom each year there are approximately 45 500 preterm babies born, and in the United States, something like 250 000. A few are born very early and may weigh as little as 600 grammes (1 lb 5 oz). The earlier a baby is born the less his appearance matches that of the normal term baby. In spite of the fact that the heavier and more mature the baby, the better the chances of his healthy survival, almost every neonatal intensive care unit can claim some successes with babies of very low birth weight and gestational ages of less than 27 weeks.

What preterm and small for gestational age babies look like

Even the most immature baby of 25 weeks or so has a normal body form right down to the smallest of finger-nails and toes. However, the more immature and preterm a baby is, the less he resembles the baby his parents had expected. His skin is thin, even transparent, and it may be easy to see blood-vessels beneath it. Skin coloration can vary dramatically from moment to moment from pink to very pale. Babies of black parents may initially have quite pale complexions, but their skin becomes progressively pigmented with age.

A preterm baby of less than 32 weeks' gestation has ribs and chest muscles that stand out because there has been insufficient time for fat tissue to accumulate beneath the skin. In a very immature baby this deficit of fat can make him look quite 'scrawny'.

The chest is also less firm than that of a more mature baby and tends to dip inwards as he breathes. Before 32 weeks the skin may be covered with a coat of fine hair (lanugo). This can be prominent on the forehead, back, shoulders, and arms, but disappears soon after birth. Small white 'pinhead' spots are commonly present over the face and upper chest. These are known as milia and are immature sweat glands that are not yet able to secrete their 'sweat' on to the skin surface.

The muscles of immature babies are weak, and this makes these babies seem quite floppy. They tend not to change position very often, and lie with arms and legs stretched out. They seem to sleep a lot of the time. The movements that such a baby does make are frequently jerky and sudden compared with the slower, more controlled, efforts of a term baby.

The umbilical cord may seem quite large compared with the size of the baby, and the junction of cord with the skin of the abdominal wall is quite prominent. The bones of the head are particularly soft and are joined by strong fibrous membranes. These are the 'soft spots'on a baby's head—the fontanelles—and move with the normal pressure changes in the head that accompany breathing and crying.

The genitalia (sex organs) are formed very early in pregnancy. However in preterm baby boys the penis may seem minute and the testes may not be fully down in the scrotum by the time the baby is born. In the preterm baby girl the inner folds (labia minora) are much larger than the outer folds (labia majora); this is just a stage in normal development.

Various physical differences, and observations made on a baby's postures and movements, enable doctors to determine the approximate maturity of an infant. Before 26 weeks' gestation there may be no breast tissue visible. The nipple develops first, and is followed by a change in the appearance of the area around it (areola). By the time a preterm baby reaches his expected date of delivery, breast tissue will have developed to a similar stage as that of a baby born at term. The tissue continues to develop normally as the child grows up. Babies of 25 weeks' gestation may have fused eyelids; these open as the baby becomes more mature.

Another feature of preterm babies is the softness of their ears. Babies born at term have cartilage in the ear which gives the ear firmness and shape. Ears of preterm babies appear wrinkled, and

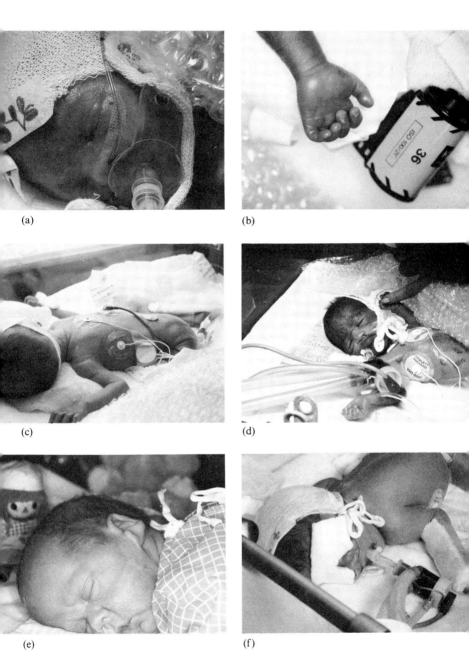

(a) A baby of 25 weeks' gestation often has fused eyelids.

(b) Although still very small at 25 weeks, fingers and nails are perfectly formed.

(c) In a preterm baby the head seems large in relation to the body and the arms and legs may be thin.

(d) With little fat beneath the skin, the ribs stand out.

(e) Owing to there being little cartilage in the ears, they may look wrinkled or folded over.

(f) The skin may have a covering of fine hair called lanugo.

Table 1.2. Fetal development

Gestational age in weeks	Behaviour and stage of tissue and organ development
6–7	Heart begins to beat. Small 'buds' where arms and legs are growing. Crown–rump length ≃ 8 mm: ├─────┤
8–9	Brain, heart, and other main organs developing rapidly. Eyes now more obvious. Ridges appear on hands and feet—the beginnings of fingers and toes. Crown–rump length ≃ 17 mm: ├─────────┤
10–14	Muscles sufficiently developed to cause movement—but not yet discernible by mother. Swallowing of amniotic fluid and passing of urine now occur.
14	Heartbeat detectable by doppler ultrasound. Crown–rump length ≃ 56 mm: ├──────────────────────────┤
15–22	Beginnings of hair, eyebrows, and eyelashes. The fine hair is called lanugo. Eyelids fused. Finger and toe-nails growing.
18–20	Kicking felt in first pregnancy; noticed earlier in subsequent pregnancies.
22–30	Vigorous movements occur. Reacts to loud noises; hiccups! Becomes covered in white, greasy 'vernix'—this protects fetus from becoming 'water-logged'. Sucking activity now visible during ultrasound scanning.
25–26	Eyelids open; eyes appear blue. Skin still paper thin; some bone now replacing cartilage in the skeleton. Brain shows little detailed structural differentiation; fluid-containing ventricles are large.
30–36	Lung maturation in preparation for air breathing is advancing rapidly. Skin creases on soles of feet deepen and increase in number. Flat margin of ear becomes progressively more incurved. Cartilage begins to give rigidity to previously floppy ears.
30–36+	Nipple areola become defined. Breast tissue increases in volume beneath the nipple. Posture becomes more flexed when lying on back:

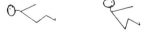

Truncal tone increases: Less head lag on pulling to sit.

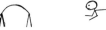

Increasing extension of neck and spine when suspended prone.

may fold over when the baby lies on them. By the equivalent of term a baby's ears are firmer and have a normal appearance.

The major differences between various gestations are indicated in Table 1.2. By the time they have reached toddlerhood most preterm born children are indistinguishable from their term born peers.

2
Why does preterm birth happen?

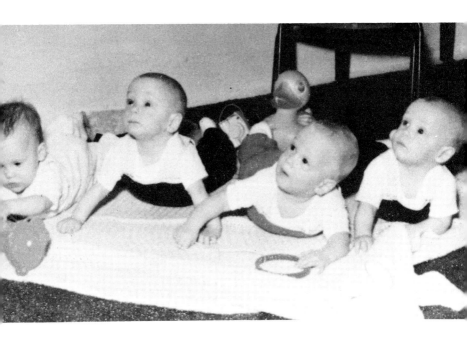

Although many factors have been found to be associated with an increased chance of a mother giving birth to her baby prematurely, the mechanisms by which preterm births are caused are usually unknown. This is why, for an individual mother who has given birth to a preterm baby, it is rarely possible to give a complete explanation about why it happened that way. The identification of a statistical association with a particular outcome, for example that of being under 17 years old and giving birth early, may shed little or no light on the mechanisms by which preterm labour occurs more frequently in this group of mothers.

None the less, obstetricians are aware of certain factors, of which some may be rectified by intervention during, or even before, the pregnancy. The aim of any such interventions is to take a pregnancy safely towards term. When there is no obvious reason for preterm birth, or when there is an unexpected emergency necessitating delivery, intervention may not be possible.

Risk factors

Table 2.1 shows a list of some of the factors that have been found to be associated with giving birth to a preterm baby. In most cases it is unclear why an association exists, but when one or more of these is present there is a statistically increased risk. Even so a mother with one, or even several of these factors, is still likely to have her baby born at term.

Some of the items listed are associated with well recognized medical consequences (e.g. smoking, alcoholism, drug addiction). What is common to all of them is some degree of stress; this may affect a mother, and her pregnancy less directly. There is debate as to whether severe psychological stress alone can in some circumstances initiate preterm labour, but there is little evidence in normal pregnancies that sexual activity does. Table 2.2 shows a list of other factors which many parents worry about and sometimes believe may have been responsible for the preterm birth of their baby. There is no good evidence that any of them is a cause. Even when obviously sudden events occur, the mechanisms by which they bring about the onset of labour is uncertain.

A good example of where an event may precipitate preterm labour is premature rupture of the membranes. These form the amniotic sac (bag of waters) in which the baby grows. Rupture can

Table 2.1. Some factors associated with preterm delivery

Previous preterm birth
Multiple pregnancy
Teenage pregnancy (under 17)
Becoming pregnant within three months of giving birth
Previous termination of pregnancy
Low maternal weight (less than 45 kg)
Maternal short stature (less than 160 cm)
Poor maternal nutrition
Poor weight gain in pregnancy
Heart disease
Infection of the urinary tract in pregnancy (cystitis)
Major illness or operation during the pregnancy
Separation of the placenta
Single or unsupported parent; divorced
Manual occupation of baby's father
Low socio-economic status of baby's mother
Heavy smoking by mother
Alcoholism in mother
Drug addiction of mother
Long stressful journeys
? Sexual activity
? Death of close relative, bereavement, or psychological stress

Table 2.2. Some factors *not* usually considered to cause preterm birth

Housework
A small fall
Climbing stairs
Continuing to work beyond 28 weeks—if physically non-demanding and psychologically non-stressful
Lifting other children
Travelling on short plane journey
Jogging

occur before the onset of contractions and labour pains, and quite a lot of the 'liquor' (fluid) surrounding the baby may gradually drain away. There is some evidence to support the idea that in certain mothers the membranes may be weaker than usual. Such speculations, however, lack proof and the mechanisms are too poorly understood at present to influence the management of the pregnancy.

If the cervix (the narrow neck at the outlet of the uterus) opens up in early pregnancy, the membranes may bulge through and then rupture. Mothers in whom this is likely to occur may be identified by having had two or more previous mid-trimester miscarriages or preterm births. Intervention in a further pregnancy may be possible if this cause of preterm labour is suspected; a special stitch can be inserted around the opening of the cervix—rather like a purse-string—before dilatation has become advanced (a Shirodkar suture or McDonald stitch). Some additional weeks of pregnancy may be gained in this way.

Intervention for the safety of mother and baby

A different category of preterm births is that in which delivery is brought about by deliberate (elective) obstetric intervention for the benefit of the mother, her baby, or both of them. Maternal high blood pressure (hypertension), kidney disease, an excess of fluid around the baby (polyhydramnios), and a pregnancy complicated by anaemia in the baby due to a mother's immune response to the baby's differing blood group, are all situations in which obstetricians may decide to deliver the baby prematurely. Other circumstances where they may intervene are those where a baby is showing signs of distress, or is growing at a poor rate, when there has been prolonged rupture of the membranes with the risk of infection reaching the baby, or when there is bleeding from the placenta. When a mother is pregnant with more than one baby it may be necessary to deliver her babies a few weeks early, particularly if she is expecting triplets or quads.

An unfortunate cause of preterm birth is the misjudgement of the maturity (gestational age) of the baby. This happens when labour is induced, or when a Caesarean section is carried out electively to bring about the delivery of a baby who is thought to be at term, but who in fact turns out to be preterm. This reflects the persisting difficulty of accurately dating some pregnancies, particularly when a mother comes late to antenatal care.

3

Preterm birth

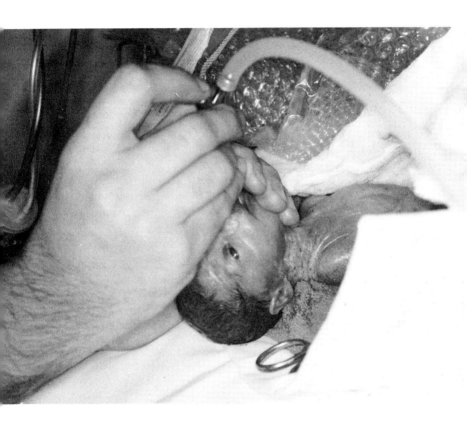

Decisions about delivery

The well-being and condition of a baby at the moment of birth greatly influences the nature and severity of the problems that can occur in the newborn period. This is why discussions between obstetricians and paediatricians before a baby's birth are necessary in helping both mother and baby come through this difficult time successfully. Talking the situation over with parents makes them aware of the options being considered for them and their baby, and provides them with an opportunity to express their own views.

Several different courses of action are possible. They mainly depend on the maturity of the baby, on the way the baby is found to be lying, and on whether or not the membranes have already ruptured. If there is doubt about the maturity of the baby, and in particular doubt about whether the lungs are going to be able to function adequately without special assistance, delivery may be delayed. A small volume of the fluid surrounding the baby can be taken by amniocentesis for chemical analysis to assess lung maturity, and the obstetrician may decide to give corticosteroid medication (e.g. Betamethasone) to the mother. The steroid crosses the placenta to the baby and, at early gestations, may enhance the maturity of the baby's lungs. In some circumstances it is not safe to delay delivery, or to give steroids, and then the newborn baby is more likely to require breathing support. The use of steroids has had an important effect on reducing the frequency and severity of the respiratory problems associated with lung immaturity in girls but probably has little effect on boys.

What happens when preterm birth threatens?

Obstetric management is generally directed towards helping a pregnancy last for as great a proportion of the normal full-term gestation period as possible, provided that the course of action will not result in a greater risk to mother or baby than early delivery. Even a week or two gained at early gestations (26–28 weeks) may have a profound effect on the outcome for the baby.

Rupture of the membranes

About 20 per cent of all mothers giving birth prematurely have a rupture of the membranes before the onset of labour (premature rupture of membranes). With this main barrier to the outside environment broken, bacteria may ascend and cause infection of the membranes (amnionitis), of the amniotic fluid, and even of the baby. Sometimes a sample of the fluid surrounding the baby is taken to determine whether infection is present. If infection of the amniotic fluid is found, energetic use of antibiotics and early delivery are indicated. When there is no infection, delaying the delivery gives time for the baby to mature further. But opinions differ about the length of time it is safe to leave a mother when the membranes have ruptured, so each mother, and her pregnancy, have to be considered individually. If it is decided to proceed with delivery drugs may be used to initiate or augment existing uterine contractions (e.g. oxytocin).

Bleeding

Bleeding from the placenta poses a threat to the baby, although it is usually the mother's, rather than the baby's, blood that is lost. Bleeding may be due to a partial breakdown of the area where the placenta is attached to the uterus. As the placenta separates (placental abruption), the exchange of oxygen and carbon dioxide between the baby and mother becomes compromised because the surface area available for exchange is reduced. If severe, the life of the baby may be at risk due to the deterioration in these essential functions. Partial separation of the placenta may trigger uterine contractions by causing the release of chemicals (prostaglandins) which increase the irritability of the uterine muscle. A decision may have to be made as to whether to deliver the baby by an emergency Caesarean section operation.

Bleeding can also occur if the placenta is low-lying—that is close to the outlet from the uterus (placenta praevia). As the lower part of the uterus lengthens in late pregnancy, separation of small areas of the placenta can occur. This cause of bleeding is often less serious and a watchful approach, with complete bed-rest in hospital, may be recommended. However, if the placenta is actually positioned so that it partly or completely obstructs the way out for the baby delivery by Caesarean section may be necessary, but not as an emergency unless the bleeding is severe.

The baby's position

The earlier in pregnancy that labour starts the more room a baby has, and the more likely he is to be lying in a breech position with feet or buttocks first. Normally a first baby adopts a cephalic (head down) position sometime between 30 and 34 weeks, but a subsequent baby may not 'turn' until later in gestation. If a baby seems to be in an 'unfavourable' position for normal birth, such as in a breech or transverse lie position (horizontally across the uterus), the decision may be made to go ahead with a Caesarean Section. Attempts to change a baby's position by external manipulation (version) are sometimes considered.

Spontaneous preterm labour

For the mother whose preterm labour starts spontaneously and for no apparent reason, the most disconcerting aspect is that the low back pains, or 'stomach cramps', she experiences may not be recognized as being caused by uterine contractions. It may not even have occurred to her that she *could* go into early labour, and so the pains may be attributed to constipation, a stomach upset, or pregnancy back-ache—even by her doctor. She may then arrive at hospital in an advanced stage of labour, by which time any treatment to inhibit the process is likely to be ineffective or even undesirable.

Provided that such a stage has not been reached, various measures may be adopted in an attempt to arrest the labour. Some of the options are outlined in Table 3. The policies and drugs which are used to stop labour will differ between centres, and between individual obstetricians; the table is therefore necessarily oversimplified.

Attempts at suppression of early labour with β agonist-type drugs are widely practised (e.g. Salbutamol, Ritodrine, etc.). The objective may be to gain 24–48 hours so that the 'glucocorticoid' (steroid) hormone, when given to a mother, may have time to enhance the maturity of the baby's lungs or, in the very preterm pregnancy, to gain more time before birth by stopping labour altogether.

Table 3.1 Outline of some aspects of the management of preterm labour

---

28–32 completed weeks

No rupture of membranes

Suppression of labour for 24 hours or longer
1. Treat cause of preterm labour if identifiable and appropriate, e.g. infection
2. Bed Rest
3. Depress uterine muscle activity
   (a) intravenous β agonist drug
   (b) (intravenous alcohol)
Enhancement of baby's lung maturation—for consideration
1. Glucocorticoid hormone for 48 hours
2. ? repeat at 7–10 day intervals

Ongoing evaluation of the baby's well-being and of risk/benefit ratio of delaying birth longer if feasible
1. Infection monitoring
2. Cardiotocography (fetal heart rate monitoring)
3. Fetal growth assessments

33–34 completed weeks

---

1. Amniocentesis to evaluate fetal lung maturation.
   Action: suppress labour if lungs immature

34–37 completed weeks

Allow labour to continue, or induce labour if membranes have ruptured.

Transfer for delivery

When the baby is estimated to be less than 32 weeks gestation, the mother may be advised to agree to being transferred to a regional centre specializing in preterm deliveries and newborn care. Some specialists feel this offers the best chance for mother and child. Alternatively, the baby may be transferred following birth if needing intensive care.

Monitoring in labour

Checking on a preterm baby's condition throughout labour is now recognized as being very important. Using an external monitor held in place on the mother's abdomen by a belt the heart rate of the baby can be monitored indirectly. Many doctors now prefer to monitor the baby's heart rate using a small clip attached to the baby's own scalp. In this way the baby's response to labour can be judged directly, and the presence of any 'distress' detected. Undesirable effects from the normal stress of labour are more likely if the baby is small for gestational age. A baby who is found not to be coping well with the stresses of labour can then be delivered more quickly, either by use of forceps or by Caesarean section. Some obstetricians use forceps to aid 'normal' preterm vaginal deliveries.

Caesarean section

A Caesarean section is often the preferred method of delivery for a preterm baby presenting as a breech. This procedure may also be performed to deliver a very preterm baby, or where there are complications of the pregnancy or labour such as bleeding.

With an anaesthetist available, and an operating theatre prepared, this procedure can take place shortly after the decision to deliver the mother has been made. It can be carried out either under epidural anaesthesia, in which case the mother will be awake but feeling no discomfort, or under a general anaesthetic in which case she will be unconscious. Usually a lower segment (LSCS) horizontal incision is made in the uterus through a small horizontal (bikini line) skin incision, although a vertical (classical) approach may be made to deliver babies in some emergency situations, and if the pregnancy is less than 30 weeks, gestation where the lower segment of the uterus is not yet formed. From the moment the surgeon begins, it can be as few as four minutes before the baby is born, though the stitching up takes rather longer.

Mothers' feelings at the time

Regardless of the way their baby is born many mothers feel cheated by a preterm birth. Surprised to find themselves in labour, they are then shocked and worried because things have not turned out as they, and their partner, expected. A mother whose labour has been stopped, or delayed, using drugs, may find herself in a state of uneasy surprise, if not acute anxiety. She may also be disturbed by side-effects such as nausea, palpitations, and tremulousness, which are commonly associated with the use of β agonist drugs.

Some mothers in preterm labour experience relatively little pain and often those who deliver without much assistance find it hard to describe the moment of birth with any excitement. 'The baby just slipped out', 'it wasn't the hard work I had expected', and 'it didn't really feel like having a baby', are comments that mothers have made about the birth of their preterm babies. For others it is a painful experience; they may not have been prepared for the fact that the obstetrician looking after them may try to limit the amount of pain-relieving drugs used during labour. This is because a small immature baby has more difficulty in metabolizing (breaking down) and excreting these drugs, which may therefore have some harmful effects.

Birth and afterwards

Undesirable effects of the normal stresses of labour and birth are more likely in a preterm than a term baby. This is why the number of interventions (e.g. monitoring) used by the obstetric team tends to be high, and what is called 'active management' is practised.

One or more paediatricians are usually present in the delivery room or operating theatre when a preterm baby is born. Their aim is to ensure the newborn baby's safety and well-being until a decision is made on whether he needs to be transferred to the baby unit. It is common for small babies to have difficulty in establishing regular and adequate breathing, and in getting enough oxygen into their blood. This is vital for the normal functioning of the heart, brain, and other organs. Various factors, including the stress experienced during labour, and pain-killing drugs given to a mother before delivery, can further reduce the baby's ability to breathe for himself. Having staff who are specially trained and quite familiar with handling very small babies, means that they can get air into the baby's lungs rapidly, no matter whether he is breathing for himself or not.

Preventing a baby from becoming cold is crucial at this time, so he will be dried to prevent evaporative heat loss, such as occurs when stepping out from a warm bath or shower. The baby is then placed on a special platform, sometimes called a resuscitaire, which has a radiant heating element above the baby to keep him warm. While lying on it his mouth and upper airway will probably be gently 'sucked out' using a soft, thin, tube to remove any mucus or fluid.

A baby's breathing can be helped by puffing with a 'bag and mask'. Alternatively, a tube can be passed through his mouth directly into the trachea (wind pipe leading to the lungs) and oxygen given through it (intubation). At this stage, if a baby's condition is stable, and no further respiratory support needed, a mother who is awake may have a chance to see and touch her baby, and possibly hold him. For other parents who are not so lucky it may be days or even weeks before they can cuddle their baby and inspect him thoroughly in the way that most parents of full-term babies like to do. If a baby cannot safely have the breathing tube removed he will be immediately transferred to the baby unit for special or intensive care. This transfer is carried out using a special transport incubator, just as occurs with journeys between hospitals, and during transfer full support and 'ventilation' of the baby's lungs can be continued if necessary. The baby may also be wrapped in a silver foil 'swaddler' for the trip to further reduce cooling.

However brief the first glimpse of their baby may be, it can be a very rewarding, if anxious moment for the parents. Undoubtedly, the most distressing situation for parents will be one in which a baby has to be moved to intensive care before his mother has woken up after a general anaesthetic. A father's role in accompanying his baby to the neonatal unit, and the reassurance that he can shortly give to the baby's mother are important, and the value must not be underestimated. Every effort should be made to involve a father initially, both for his own benefit and the part he can play helping the mother cope with this upsetting situation.

Unexpected preterm birth at home

Because preterm labour contractions may go unnoticed, or be passed off as something unimportant, a small proportion of mothers having preterm babies accidentally give birth at home. If this occurs the baby, and particularly his head, should be wrapped up warmly and the emergency ambulance services contacted immediately. It is probably best to leave the umbilical cord uncut and untied. There are preterm babies who do well in spite of such an inauspicious beginning.

4

Special care for preterm babies

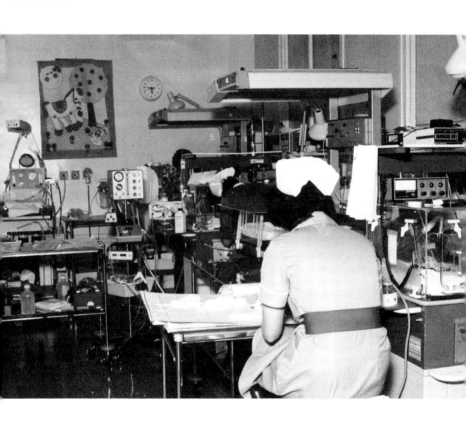

High risk mothers and babies

The establishment of centres specializing in the care of mothers with high risk pregnancies and of their newborn, often preterm, babies, has its origins in the 1960s, for it was then that the possible preventive role of providing special care for high risk mothers was recognized. The mothers were those considered to be at risk of giving birth prematurely, those with unexpected complications of pregnancy, and those who were actually in preterm labour. This awareness of the possible benefits of increased care has led to changes in the regional organization of care provision for such mothers, and for their infants.

The need for specialization, both in obstetrics and neonatal care, brought about the development of regional centres, which in the UK are located on the basis of the National Health Service geographically designated regions (level III centres in the USA). Other hospital units also having the capability for carrying out intensive newborn care have been provided, although lesser degrees of provision are to be found in most district hospitals (level II and level I capabilities in the USA). This rationalization has been necessary in view of the restricted resources available.

Since the beginnings of intensive care there has been a steady fall in the mortality rate of the most at risk preterm newborns and a marked reduction in severe handicap amongst the very low birthweight survivors (less than 1500 g or $3\frac{1}{4}$ lb.). An improved survival amongst babies needing ventilator assistance because of immaturity of their lungs has also been noted. In the early 1960s very few babies survived this disorder if it was severe. Now over 90 per cent of these babies, if born weighing more than 1 kg (2 lb 3 oz) at birth, and requiring assistance with their breathing, would be expected to live, due to the improvements in newborn care. As a consequence intensive care for the newborn has become increasingly available.

Intensive care

The division between intensive and special care is rather an artificial one. It is generally accepted that full intensive (tertiary) care provision is dependent upon a unit having the necessary, and now extensive, equipment, medical expertise, specialized investigational facilities, and a very high standard of nursing skill. Such care must be able to be given for long periods when necessary. The need for social worker and health visitor involvement, and support, is also apparent in view of the many problems experienced by families with a baby that has been born too soon.

Many district (community) hospitals have facilities for 'special care', without necessarily being able to provide prolonged highly sophisticated support. Such units would expect to transfer out those babies needing the more intensive forms of treatment. Research is usually carried out at the major referral centres on many different aspects of prematurity and its problems; it is from the widespread application of the findings of this reasearch that continued progress is being made.

Other kinds of care

No matter how good the team of doctors and nurses at an intensive care centre might be, if the outcome for a baby and his family is to

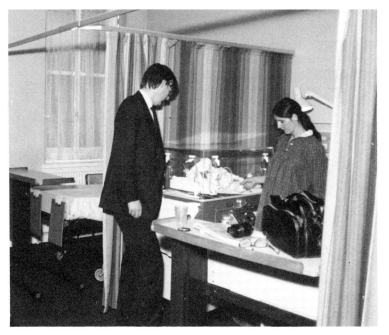

A well preterm baby can be looked after on a postnatal ward if kept warm in an incubator.

be optimal local or peripheral units must be able to provide adequate resuscitation and initial treatment from birth. This must include a sufficiently warm environment to prevent the baby losing body heat before he is transferred. Ventilatory support (specialized breathing assistance) should also be available in the short term to ensure that the harmful effects of inadequate breathing or insufficient oxygenation of the baby are prevented.

Some 10-20 per cent of newborn babies are given some form of specialized care (intermediary), and about a third of those need the intensive care such as that usually provided by a regional centre (tertiary care).

In some hospitals a small baby, who is otherwise well, may be nursed in an incubator beside his mother so that she can help care for him. This is sometimes referred to as 'transitional care', for it represents a cross between the neonatal unit and the normal post-natal ward. In a very few hospitals, which are perhaps pointing the way for the future, 'mother and baby' rooms are incorporated into the neonatal unit so that mothers are not separated from their babies. This enables a mother to be close to her baby even though the baby may be quite ill and receiving intensive care.

Transfer of the baby to an intensive care unit

There are usually extra medical staff in the delivery room to help when a preterm baby is expected. The 'transport team' from the referral centre, comprising a doctor experienced in the care of such babies, and a specially trained nurse, may also be there. Alternatively, this team may only be called in if the baby develops problems.

Some units have a vehicle that has been specifically designed for transfer, while others rely on a 'transport incubator' which can easily be put in a normal ambulance. The use of a helicopter or plane is rare in the United Kingdom, although these forms of transport are quite often used in North America and Australia due to the much greater distances involved.

Modes of transferring 'at risk' preterm babies are still needed, in spite of the increasing number of mothers who are being transferred to specialized centres before having their babies. This is because it is not always desirable, or safe, to transfer a mother before delivery for either social or medical reasons.

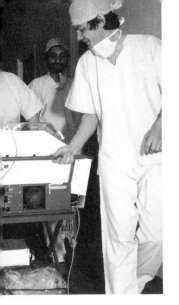
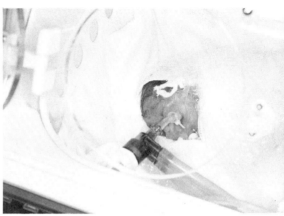

The transport incubator is specially designed to enable full care, including breathing support, warmth, monitoring, and fluid administration, to be given during the transfer from the delivery suite or for much longer journeys between hospitals. The baby is often wrapped in a silver 'foil' sheet to reduce heat loss.

When a baby needs to be transferred to a different hospital soon after birth, arrangements are often made for the mother to be moved at the same time or shortly afterwards. She can then receive her early postnatal care in the obstetric department at the referral centre. This is of course only possible when the hospital to which the baby has been moved has its own maternity department; some neonatal units are located in children's hospitals without such facilities. The advantages to a mother and baby of being together are considerable. Such an arrangement will reduce a mother's anxiety and enable her to participate in the early care of her baby. The baby's father can then be with both of them rather than having the added stress, and wasted time and money, involved in visiting two separate hospitals. Some of the problems that result from family separations are discussed in Chapter 6.

None would deny that the transfer of a baby, or a mother, can create difficulties and disrupt family life a great deal, but one has to accept that the emergence of special centres of excellence has been central to the improved results of intensive care for newborns that have taken place over the last two decades.

The people providing pregnancy and family-centered newborn care

Obstetricians are doctors who are responsible for the care of a mother during pregnancy, delivery, and afterwards, and may at times visit the baby unit.

Paediatricians are doctors who have had special training in the care of children and the newborn.

Neonatologists are usually doctors who are principally involved in the care of newborns. This specialty is less common in the United Kingdom then, for example, in the United States. They are available on 'stand-by' call.

Junior medical staff or residents are doctors at differing levels of special training in paediatrics and newborn care, available on 24 hour call.

Senior nursing staff. A nursing officer or superintendent may have overall management of the unit. Nurses of the 'sister' grade in an intensive care unit (tertiary care, level III centre) have usually obtained special training in neonatal care, and may previously have been in midwifery or general paediatric nursing. In North America nurse practitioners receive more intensive training which enables them to carry out many of the procedures performed by doctors in the UK.

The sister in charge co-ordinates the medical and nursing contributions to the care of babies and parents. She has a major responsibility in ensuring staff awareness of changing medical and nursing practices. Parental bewilderment due to conflicting medical and nursing viewpoints can only be avoided when there is a fully integrated team approach, and ample opportunities for communication between staff.

Nursing staff comprise state registered (SRN) or state enrolled nurses (SEN), registered sick children's nurses (RSCN) and state certified midwives (SCM) at differing levels of training and experience in the care of newborns. Nursery nurses have received training in general child care at a College of Further Education, and possess a certificate from the Nursery Nurses Examination Board.

Different grades of nursing staff can usually be distinguished by their caps, badges, or the colour of their uniforms.

Research staff. In major centres there may be researchers carrying out studies or investigating problems relating to newborn babies and their care. Examples of these are doctors, nurses, and psychologists with interest in behaviour and developmental progress, and physiologists and biochemists concerned with the many different aspects of the way the newborn body functions.

Physiotherapists (physical therapists) provide help for babies with breathing difficulties by assisting them in clearing mucus from their chests. They also advise on muscle and joint movements. Often they are the same people who have taught mothers antenatally, and advised on postnatal exercises after the birth.

Radiographers are trained in the use of X-ray equipment and visit the baby unit with a portable X-ray machine.

Social workers are specially trained individuals, one or more of whom are often directly involved in the baby unit. At some time antenatally, parents may have been introduced to at least one of the hospital's team of social workers. They can provide help and advice on problems of visiting, housing, and finance. Some parents find it helpful to talk over other more personal problems too, and when things seem difficult to cope with parents should be made aware of the availability of a social worker to help them.

Health visitors are nurses or midwives who have undergone additional training in community health education. Some neonatal units have a liaison health visitor who is familiar with the babies there. She can make contact with the family's local health visitor who will visit the family once the mother, and then the baby, are home. Health visitors give advice on child care and information to parents about health services in the community.

Psychiatrists, psychotherapists, and clinical psychologists are specifically trained to be able to deal with emotional and other psychological aspects of health. Psychiatrists are also qualified medical doctors, whereas clinical psychologists and psychotherapists complete postgraduate studies after a first degree in psychology. In the United States, hospital psychiatric services are commonly available directly, though in Britain parents who request such help may have to go through their family doctor or social worker.

Domestic staff help with the vast amounts of cleaning that have to be done.

Parents, though not strictly 'staff', have been included on this list because they have such a vital role, not simply in caring for their own baby, but also through their discussions with the staff and other parents. In some units parent groups have been formed to encourage a supportive atmosphere, and parents whose babies have previously been on the baby unit sometimes also attend.

Recognizing the staff

In many hospitals members of staff wear name badges and the different uniforms aid identification. In other units there may be a 'photo board' so that parents, and even new staff, can find out who's who without having to try and read indecipherable name tags, or be embarrassed by having to ask directly.

Primary nursing—in which total individualized care for a baby and family are provided on a continuous basis, is becoming increasingly popular in the United States. The nurse providing such care has the authority to act as chief nurse for her patient, each day, until the patient is discharged. When not present she assigns the care to secondary or associate nurses, and she is responsible for the daily reporting and communication of details concerning the patient to other disciplines. She would also be responsible for parent teaching, and for assessment of parent readiness for homecoming; she would make and co-ordinate the discharge arrangements, follow-up referrals, and community liaison. The advantage of such an approach is that it makes a staff member accountable for the quality and continuity of a baby's nursing care, and for ensuring that the family's needs are fully appreciated and met. It can lead to a much more individualized form of care with considerable staff and parental satisfaction.

No matter which system of care is being practised, it is vital that continuing critical appraisal of medical and nursing practices, based on our expanding factual knowledge, should replace the uncreative, stagnant, 'that's the way we always do it here' approach.

5

Medical care for preterm babies

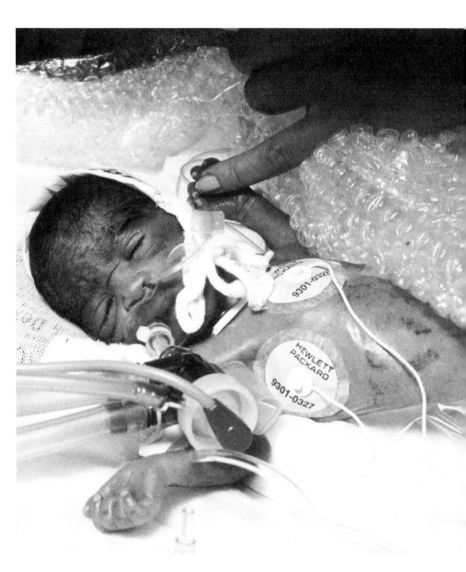

Medical equipment and procedures

Individual babies have very different needs and problems, and what can be seen going on in any baby unit will reflect these varying requirements. The equipment and techniques which have been evolved to cope with these needs are discussed in some detail in the sections that follow.

Some similar items of equipment and procedures may have been mentioned previously in Chapter 3 in relation to the care given to a preterm baby in the delivery room, or operating theatre. Because of the many and continuing improvements in neonatal care, a range of equipment designs may be in use in just one unit, and there may be considerable differences between units in the way things are done.

Problems for the preterm baby

The major practical problems for a baby who has been born too soon are related to his relative immaturity. Therefore the more immature the baby, the more troublesome the problems tend to be.

Keeping warm. Until birth the baby has been able to rely on his mother's body to supply this need. Once the baby is born he has to maintain his body temperature and prevent it from fluctuating.

Breathing adequately. In the uterus, the placenta performs the equivalent of this function, but the newborn has to breathe to obtain oxygen for himself. This activity is essential if other body systems are to work optimally.

Maintaining the correct fluid balance. While the baby is growing in his mother his body fluids are accurately maintained by the placenta. Once a baby is delivered he is subjected to external influences and may be unable to compensate adequately.

Obtaining nourishment. Before birth a baby relies on receiving nutriment via the placenta, and disposes of most waste-products in the same way. Once outside he is dependent on what he is given, and what he can absorb; his 'food' must not only be appropriate for his digestive capability, but also adequate for growth and development.

Monitoring the baby

Monitoring is the process of keeping track of vital functions using electrical devices. This begins in the delivery room, continues during transfer, and is a routine part of 'care' in the neonatal unit.

Body warmth

An unstable temperature is common in preterm babies; their temperature may rise too high (a fever or hyperthermia), or fall too low (hypothermia), due to small changes in the environment. Whereas a term baby may be able to compensate effectively, a premature baby cannot. Hypothermia causes 'cold stress', and although the baby tries to maintain his warmth by using up more oxygen and energy resources, often he does not succeed. This is because a preterm baby, as well as having little in the way of energy stores, has little fat beneath his skin to insulate him, and has a relatively large body surface from which he can lose heat. Conversely, if a preterm baby does get too warm he cannot sweat to cool himself as older babies do because his sweat glands and sweat production are not sufficiently developed. Very preterm babies can lose a lot of water through their very thin skins, and evaporation cools them rapidly. This represents a further uncontrollable source of heat loss.

Temperature measurement

Using a thermometer, a baby's temperature can be recorded from under the armpit (axillary temperature), or from just inside his rectum (rectal temperature). Often temperature is recorded continuously by means of a temperature-sensitive probe taped onto the baby's abdomen. This is linked to a visual display unit (VDU) nearby, so his temperature may be seen at a glance.

Keeping preterm babies warm

An open crib with a radiant heat source, sometimes referred to as a platform bed, is one way of nursing preterm babies, particularly small ones. Such beds (Fig. 5.1) usually have integral skin temperature monitoring, and for this two probes are placed on the baby's

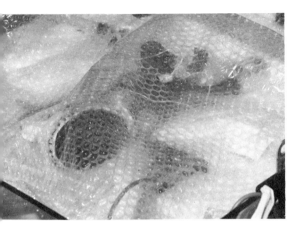
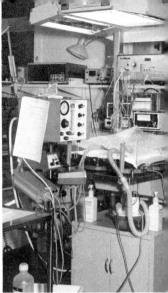

Nursing a baby on an open platform bed allows excellent access, but a covering such as bubble plastic is needed to reduce water losses through the skin.

abdomen. These are connected to a control panel and as the baby's temperature rises or falls, heat is automatically given out according to his needs. Reducing the loss of water through the skin, which is more likely in this open situation, is achieved by covering the baby with a sheet of 'bubble' plastic, 'cling-film', or other similar material. Warm, humidified, moist, air can be passed under the plastic blanket to create an atmosphere similar to that in an incubator, but with the advantage that there is better access to the baby.

An incubator is a clear plastic 'box' in which air is circulated over heater elements in the base, and then into the top where the baby lies. The heat level can be adjusted to a desired air temperature, or to keep the baby's own temperature within set limits. The air can also be humidified, and it is this that can cause the sides of the incubator to 'steam-up'. The temperature can drop when the doors or portholes are opened and so a baby may need to be covered at these times (Fig. 5.2).

A heat shield is a transparent dome that can be placed over a baby to reduce the radiant heat loss from his skin to the walls of the incubator. This happens because the sides of the incubator, being in contact with the air circulating in the room outside, are cooler than the baby.

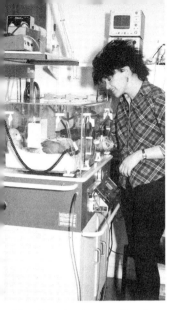
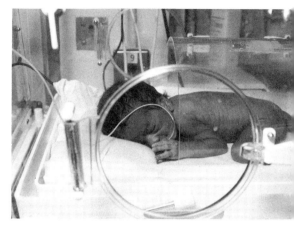

Even in an incubator, radiant heat can be lost from the baby's body to the incubator walls and an additional plastic dome, a 'heat shield', may be needed to keep the baby warm.

As a baby's size increases, and as he matures, he is better able to control his body temperature, and less temperature monitoring is needed. The incubator temperature is gradually reduced to that of room air so that he can begin to adapt to the cooler environment of a cot, or basinette, in the nursery.

The mechanics of breathing

When we breathe in we draw air, which contains oxygen (O_2), into our lungs. On breathing out, carbon dioxide (CO_2), which comes from the bloodstream, is expelled. Although a baby starts making breathing movements long before birth, breathing takes on a new significance as soon as the supply of oxygen crossing the placenta ceases at the moment of birth.

At the moment of birth a baby's lungs are filled with fluid which is displaced by the air drawn in during the baby's first breaths. The ability to inflate the lungs depends in part on the strength of the baby's respiratory (breathing) muscles, and on the stimulation they receive from his brain. In a preterm baby the wall of the chest, made up of ribs and muscles, is more flimsy than a term baby's, and so although he may make great efforts to fill his lungs with air, his chest may 'draw in', or 'recess', at every breath, instead of expanding. This is one reason why the paediatrician attending his birth may have to assist the baby's efforts by puffing with a 'bag and mask', or by passing a tube into the baby's windpipe (intubation) and then inflating the lungs directly with oxygen and air (Fig. 5.3).

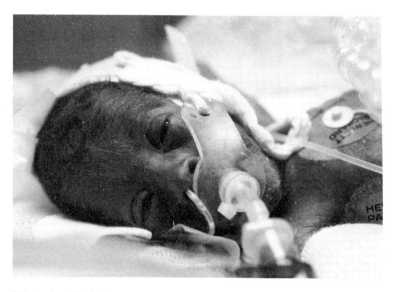

This intubated baby has a tube passing through his mouth and into the trachea (windpipe); it is held in place by a gauze bonnet tied to the plastic tube holder. Although needing respiratory support, he is aware of people near him.

How easily a baby breathes after birth also depends on whether he is sleeping lightly or deeply. In light, or 'dream' sleep, when a baby's eyelids may be seen to move, the muscles of the chest wall are less active and his breathing may become less well co-ordinated. A baby may also at times partially close off his larynx at the entry to his windpipe so that just below the margin of his rib cage his tummy can be seen to dip inwards at every inspiratory (breathing in) effort. This is because the pathway for the airflow to his lungs has become obstructed. During light sleep a baby is more likely to pause between bursts of more rapid breathing. The pauses tend to be longer in light than in deep sleep, and this pattern is referred to as 'periodic' breathing.

Babies breathe naturally through their noses. If the nose becomes blocked they may sneeze to clear it but, unlike adults, some do not automatically open their mouths to breathe when this happens. The control of breathing is less well organised the more immature the baby. The pauses may be prolonged, and are known as 'apnoeic episodes' or apnoeas; they may occur quite frequently.

Monitors and other means of detecting problems

Electrical and pressure sensitive alarm systems are used to record a baby's breathing rate (the number of times that he breathes each minute) and to monitor the pattern, and detect apnoeic episodes. If a prolonged pause occurs the alarm sounds and immediately draws the nurse's attention to the baby. These alarm systems can be a mattress under the baby which detects the movements of breathing, or a small pressure disc placed on the baby's abdomen. (Fig. 5.4).

During apnoeic pauses, and sometimes during ineffectual 'breathing' the baby's heart rate slows (bradycardia). This can also

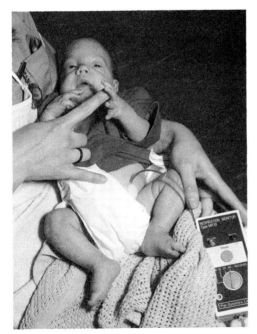

Respiration is monitored in several ways; apnoeic episodes in larger babies can be detected by a pressure-sensitive disc taped to the lower abdomen and attached to its portable alarm box.

activate an alarm that is pre-set to sound if the rate falls below specified limits. The monitor is connected to the baby by means of stickers on the chest, or by small bands around the arms and legs. If a lead becomes disconnected, or the contact between the sticker and chest becomes inadequate, the alarm will sound. Even small babies can pull them off! Transient high or low rates frequently accompany crying and unco-ordinated 'dream sleep' breathing. As a baby gets older the pattern and efficiency of his breathing mature, and these aids are no longer needed.

An apnoeic episode can usually be stopped by stimulating the baby with a flick to his hand or foot; medications, such as caffeine or theophylline derivatives, can be given to reduce the frequency of these episodes. Providing a slight 'stretch' stimulus to the baby's lungs, by giving air at raised pressure, can reduce their occurrence (see the section on the use of CPAP later in this chapter).

Oxygen and carbon dioxide

The levels of oxygen and carbon dioxide in the blood are normally maintained within narrow limits by changes in the rate, depth, and pattern of our breathing. This enables the organs of the body to function in an optimal physiological environment. The air that we breathe contains 21 per cent oxygen, but higher concentrations can be achieved in an incubator, within a box placed over the baby's head (a head box), with a mask over his face, or by using a venti-lator. The 'gases' can be humidified with water vapour to help loosen the mucus in the baby's airways. The actual amount of oxygen given is decided on the basis of measurements of oxygen in the baby's blood.

The use of arterial lines

Knowing the levels of oxygen and carbon dioxide in blood enables the medical staff caring for a preterm baby to decide when extra oxygen or breathing support is needed, and when the amount of support may be reduced. The use of fine catheters (flexible plastic tubes) which can be passed through one of the arteries in the umbilical cord to the descending aorta (the main blood-vessel from the heart to the lower limbs) can help greatly with monitoring the oxygen and carbon dioxide levels. Short cannulae (semi-rigid tubes) can also be inserted directly into an artery at the wrist (where the pulse can be felt), or at the ankle. Some catheters have an oxygen sensor at their tip, and others emit light of defined wavelengths which is then reflected back up them from the blood moving past the tip. Both types enable the amount of oxygen present in the blood to be monitored continuously. Blood samples can also be withdrawn at intervals without disturbing the baby for the measurement of oxygen, carbon dioxide, and blood 'acids' in a 'blood gas analyser'.

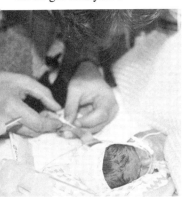
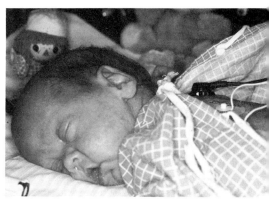

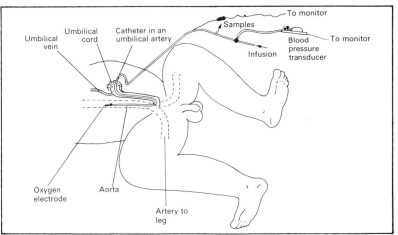

The oxygen level can be measured in a blood sample drawn directly from an artery, as here from a radial line, or by measuring the oxygen passing through warmed skin using a probe and monitor. The monitor gives a readout of the 'transcutaneous oxygen' (TcO_2) level. The oxygen level can also be monitored continuously using an umbilical artery catheter with an oxygen-sensitive electrode at its tip, as shown in the diagram.

Transcutaneous (skin) oxygen monitoring

In babies who are recovering, or who do not need a lot of support with their breathing, the oxygen and carbon dioxide levels can be monitored less intrusively using special sensors placed on the skin. These sensors contain a warming device which promotes dilatation (opening up) of the blood-vessels in the skin, and therefore a good flow of blood, so that oxygen or carbon dioxide can diffuse through the skin to the sensor more easily, and be measured. Intermittent blood samples are taken to check the readings from the skin monitor, but these cannot give an immediate indication of a change in a baby's oxygen requirements as continuous monitoring methods do.

The use of CPAP

Providing air or oxygen at a slightly increased pressure is known as CPAP (continuous positive airway pressure). This is achieved by means of nasal 'prongs', a nasal tube, a face mask, or an endotracheal tube. The positive pressure provides a 'stretch' stimulus to the lungs during a baby's spontaneous breathing, and can reduce, or abolish, apnoeic episodes; it also helps prevent the collapse of the tiny air spaces and air passages in the lungs as the baby breathes out, and helps 'stabilize' the chest wall—particularly during light sleep—in preterm babies.

Maturity of the lungs

On breathing out a small volume of air is normally left in the lungs. This is partly due to the presence of a group of materials lining the small airspaces of the lungs called surfactants, which prevent the spaces collapsing—rather as 'bubble bath' solutions stabilize bubbles in water. Some preterm babies do not have enough surfactant during the first days of life and develop progressive collapse of the airspaces. This condition is known as respiratory distress syndrome (RDS) but may sometimes be referred to as hyaline membrane disease (HMD). The lungs become very stiff, and the surface area for oxygen and carbon dioxide exchange becomes insufficient for normal levels of gases in the blood to be maintained. Extra oxygen is then given, and treatment aimed at keeping the baby's lungs expanded and free of collapse is begun.

Mechanical ventilation

When simpler supportive measures like CPAP are not enough, as shown by deteriorating levels of oxygen or carbon dioxide in the bloodstream, by respiratory fatigue, or by apnoea, intubation of the baby will be carried out. In this procedure an endotracheal tube is passed through the nose or mouth into the trachea (windpipe) and a machine called a 'ventilator' is used to supplement, or completely take over, breathing for the baby (Fig. 5.6).

Most modern ventilators (respirators) provide a background of continuous gas flow of desired oxygen content with superimposed 'puffs' of positive pressure to inflate the lungs. Following this inspiratory (or breathing in) phase, a pause allows the inspired gases to leave the lungs. During the expiratory (or breathing out) phase, a positive pressure may be maintained in the airway to reduce the chance of the small airspaces in the lungs collapsing. The rate of breathing can be pre-set as can the peak (highest) pressure delivered to the baby's lungs.

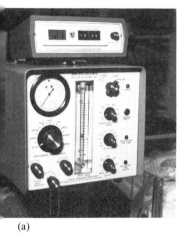
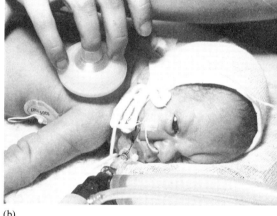

(a)   (b)

(a) The ventilator controls enable the breathing rate, pressures, and oxygen level and flow to be accurately monitored and adjusted according to the baby's changing requirements.

(b) 'Vibrations' applied to the chest wall help loosen the secretions in the lungs so that they can be cleared by suction through the endotracheal tube of a ventilated baby.

In some neonatal intensive care units muscle relaxants are used when babies are put on ventilators. By temporarily using drugs to paralyse, or to sedate a baby who is on a ventilator, it may be possible to improve the level of oxygen in the blood and control the level of carbon dioxide better in the more severely affected infants.

In 'weaning' a baby off mechanical ventilation partial support can be given by providing a continuous flow of gas with a reduced number of assisted breaths per minute (intermittent mandatory ventilation, IMV). Some babies may need more help than others to come off the ventilator, and some do better with a period on CPAP following ventilation. Sometimes medication, such as theophylline, is given at this time to help reduce periodic breathing.

Following ventilation a few babies go through a time of needing extra oxygen to breathe. Sometimes this requirement can last for weeks, or even months, and is associated with changes in the structure of the lungs called bronchopulmonary dysplasia (BPD).

Mouth suction

Preterm babies born before 32–34 weeks' gestation do not have a well developed cough reflex, protective laryngeal reflex (choking response), or co-ordinated swallowing pattern. Saliva therefore accumulates in the mouth and may be inhaled into the lungs without the choking or coughing which would normally prevent this from happening. These babies may need frequent gentle mouth 'suctioning' or 'sucking out' to clear away mucus and saliva. This is usually done with a soft, fine, tube.

Chest drains

If an air leak develops from the airspaces in a lung so that air begins to collect in the lung tissues, or between the lung itself and the wall of the chest, the function of the compressed underlying lung is impaired, and the air may have to be removed. A collection of air between lung and chest wall is called a pneumothorax, and is detected on an X-ray of the chest, or by applying a bright light to the outside of the chest wall (transillumination). Some babies have more than one of these leaks, which can occur at different times during treatment. Under the effect of a local anaesthetic a

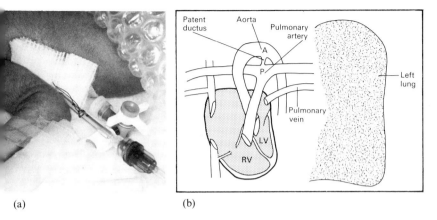

Patent ductus | Aorta | Pulmonary artery
P
A
LV
RV
Pulmonary vein
Left lung

(a)   (b)

(a) The narrow tube, passed between two ribs, is draining air from a pneumothorax caused by an air-leak from the baby's lung.

(b) The ductus arteriosus, connecting the main arteries from the heart, may remain open (patent) in a preterm baby.

pneumothorax can be drained by passing one or more tubes into the air pocket that has collected. Gentle suction is maintained until the air leak has sealed off, and the tube is then removed (Fig. 5.7). The small scars at the sites of tube insertion fade as the child gets older, and frequently become invisible.

The heart and circulation of the blood

In addition to changes associated with the stimuli to breathe, and to maintain a normal body temperature, birth brings with it changes in the heart and blood-vessels (cardiovascular system). Before birth the baby's heart has to pump blood to all parts of his body as well as through the placenta so that oxygen may be taken up and waste-products eliminated. After birth there is a marked increase in blood flow to the lungs, ensuring that the oxygen that is breathed in with a baby's first gasps is taken up efficiently by the blood. Before birth a baby's lungs have been maturing but they have not been involved in oxygen exchange; oxygen reaches the baby by means of umbilical (cord) circulation, and the level of oxygen is dependent on the mother's breathing, and on her placental blood supply. In an unborn baby, therefore, blood largely bypasses the lungs, going through a channel running between the main blood-vessel to the lungs, and the major artery of the body; this channel is the *Ductus arteriosus*. The *Ductus arteriosus* closes functionally in the first day or so after birth, and eventually becomes obliterated. However in preterm babies it may remain 'patent' (open) for much longer—a persisting patent *Ductus arteriosus* (PDA).

Heart murmurs

If blood flow becomes turbulent as it passes through a persisting open ductus, through a narrowed valve within the heart, or through any narrow obstruction, this turbulence can be detected as a 'murmur', which is rather like the noise of disturbed water in a fast flowing stream. Murmurs are common in newborn babies because of the many circulatory changes that go on during the first few days of life.

A patent ductus is the most common cause of a murmur in a preterm baby and it frequently closes spontaneously as the baby get older. Occasionally treatment is needed, but this is more likely to take the form of medication than surgery nowadays. The operation involves closing-off this channel which lies outside the heart.

Blood transfusions, blood flow, and blood-pressure

Some preterm babies may need one or more transfusions of blood at some time during their stay in hospital. Although we tend to think of blood as one substance it has many constituents, and a baby may be given 'whole' blood, or just some of its component parts. The red blood cells that carry oxygen, the white cells that fight infections, the platelets that help stop bleeding, and the plasma, the fluid in which they are all suspended, can each be given separately by being infused into a vein over a period of a few hours.

The pressure at which blood is maintained in the circulation is called the blood-pressure (BP). It can be monitored directly from an artery using a special pressure-sensitive transducer, or else indirectly using a pressure cuff and an ultrasound probe. The probe detects the return of blood flow once the cuff is deflated, converting the echoes reflected from the flowing blood into audible sound-waves. Whichever method is used, obtaining information about a

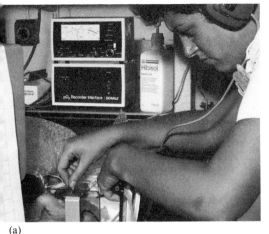

(a) Using a doppler ultrasound probe, the nurse is measuring the baby's blood pressure by listening to the sound waves reflected from the blood flowing in an artery.

(b) and (c) A baby can be soothed during the taking of a blood sample by giving her something to suck on and by holding her close.

(a)

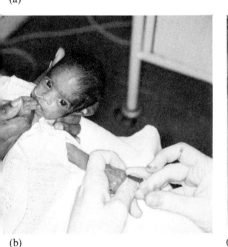

(b)

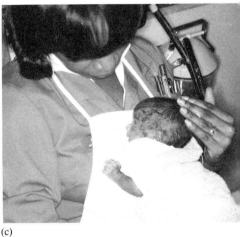

(c)

preterm baby's blood-pressure is very important because a normal blood-pressure is needed to ensure an adequate flow of blood around the body, and hence a good supply of oxygen to all the tissues. Occasionally drugs may be given to try and improve blood flow to certain organs, such as the lungs or kidneys.

Anaemia

Anaemia is a condition in which there is a lower than normal level of oxygen-carrying pigment in the blood (a low haemoglobin). The cut-off level for defining anaemia varies according to gestational and postnatal age. In babies that have been born too soon, anaemia results from having too few red blood cells to carry the haemoglobin, but the precise causes of this are not well understood.

Blood transfusions are given as treatment to increase ,the oxygen-carrying capacity of the blood, and so improve many of the baby's functions and activities. Following correction of this condition, improved feeding and fewer apnoeic episodes may be noted. Some babies, born at less than 30 weeks' gestation need several small 'top up' transfusions, and very immature babies may need them daily early on.

Taking blood samples

To make appropriate changes in therapy it is essential to monitor the levels of the different blood components in a preterm baby. Blood samples can be obtained painlessly from previously sited arterial catheters, or cannulae, or, with mild discomfort, through a needle introduced into a vein. Some very small samples can be obtained from pricking a baby's heel; this explains the sticking plasters often seen on a baby's heels.

Infusions

Fluids can be given to a baby by infusing them directly into an artery or a vein. This means that either a catheter, or a cannula (short plastic tube), or a needle, has to be sited in the chosen blood-vessel. The fluids are then infused by a syringe driver or infusion pump, the rate of infusion being pre-set and accurately controlled. Nutrients, medications, minerals, and fluids, including blood, can be given in this way. (Fig. 5.9) Though the presence of a catheter or cannula does not seem to cause discomfort getting them into position may do so; should they become displaced, or the blood-vessel blocked (thrombosed), swelling and discomfort is likely to occur as the fluid spreads beneath the skin. When it is not

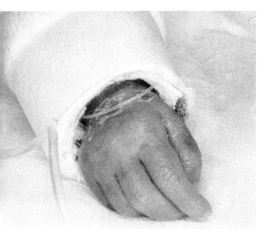

Total intravenous nutrition can be provided through a very fine tube passed into a vein and up into the right atrium of the heart where the nutrients are diluted by the high flow of blood there. Accidental withdrawal of the tube is prevented by securely wrapping up the limb in tube gauze.

possible to rely on absorption from an immature digestive system then venous routes of administration are invaluable.

Other effects of immaturity

The liver is the largest abdominal organ and performs many essential biochemical functions: releasing sugar into the blood, synthesizing proteins, metabolizing drugs, and eliminating waste-materials.

In preterm babies the liver may not produce enough blood-clotting factors or protein for the baby's needs and these may have to be provided by infusions. The dosages of some antibiotics and other medications may have to be adjusted according to the liver's ability to eliminate them. Too little production of a protein, albumin, can result in a baby becoming 'puffy' or oedematous to look at, particularly the arms and legs and around the eyes. Low levels of clotting factors may predispose a baby to bleeding, and the immaturity of the systems within the liver that 'breakdown' waste-products can cause the baby to become jaundiced.

Jaundice is the yellowness caused by pigment released from red blood cells as they are removed from the blood at the end of their lifespan. The pigment is called bilirubin and the mature liver changes it chemically so that it can be excreted in bile, and thereby eliminated in the stools. Immaturity of the liver cells results in a build-up of bilirubin in the bloodstream and body tissues, giving the baby a yellow colour.

The level of bilirubin can be checked by taking small blood samples from the baby, and if it continues to rise treatment can be instituted. This consists of placing the baby under white or blue 'phototherapy' lights. These do not give out ultra-violet light, as is commonly thought, but the special wavelength of the light emitted does act on the bilirubin pigment in the skin causing it to be broken down (photodegradation). To achieve maximum effect the baby's skin must be fully exposed so he will have no clothes on, perhaps not even a nappy, and will just have pads, or a mask, to shield his eyes. The lights themselves do not give off much heat and care has to be taken to keep a baby who is not in an incubator warm.

The blue lights can make a baby look a rather strange colour and parents often worry about this, as well as being concerned because their baby seems restless and cries more whilst under phototherapy lights. This is not usually because the lights themselves bother the baby, but because most babies are more contented when wrapped up snuggly. Although parents are often worried by phototherapy it usually prevents jaundice from becoming a major problem, and the treatment is frequently only needed for a few days. Occasionally it may be necessary to lower the bilirubin level

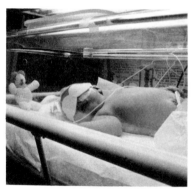

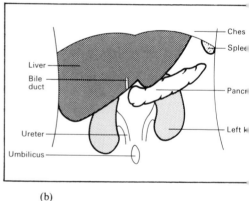

(a)   (b)

(a) The jaundiced baby having phototherapy is naked to allow maximal exposure to the lights and is kept warm by a plastic cover over his cot.

(b) Diagram showing: the *liver*, where bilirubin is conjugated and then excreted, the *pancreas*, where insulin is produced and passes into the circulation to enable sugar in the blood to be utilized, the *kidneys* where urine is produced.

more quickly by changing the baby's blood (an exchange transfusion), but nowadays most babies with jaundice need no more than phototherapy.

Exchange transfusion

If the level of bilirubin is sufficiently high, it may occasionally be necessary to 'exchange' a baby's blood with that of a donor. The particular level at which an exchange transfusion is performed will depend on the baby's gestation, his postnatal age, and whether or not he is otherwise well.

A similar procedure may be performed if a baby has too many red blood cells in the circulation (polycythaemia). Too many cells make the blood thicker and very viscous, and this causes problems (hyperviscosity syndrome). A 'dilutional' exchange is carried out in which some of the baby's blood is exchanged for albumin, plasma, or some other fluid.

The pancreas is a smaller organ adjacent to the liver and its main functions are to release the hormone insulin into the blood, and digestive enzymes and alkali into the intestine to aid food absorption. Insulin enables the glucose (sugar) in the blood to pass into body cells to meet their energy needs.

In very preterm babies neither of these functions may be adequate. Insulin may have to be given by injection (as happens for a diabetic) if the glucose in the bloodstream rises to a very high level; however the inadequate release of insulin from the pancreas is usually transient. A lack of digestive enzymes may contribute to the poor absorption of some of the constituents of the milk fed to preterm babies, but this too improves with increasing maturity.

Infections

Defences against bacteria (germs) are less well developed in a preterm baby than one who is full-term, and the early signs of infection are often unremarkable when compared with the high fever that occurs in an older child or adult. In Chapter 6 on visiting, emphasis is justifiably placed on the importance of careful hand-washing and thorough hand-drying before touching a preterm baby so as to reduce the transfer of bacteria.

In a neonatal unit many checks are routinely made for the presence of potentially infectious organisms. Swabs may be regularly taken from a baby's mouth, nose, umbilicus, and genital region, and sent for laboratory analysis. When an infection is actually suspected several additional tests may be performed in an attempt to find out exactly what the infection is, and where it is located. Urine may be collected by placing an adhesive bag over the genitals and hoping that it won't be kicked off before a specimen is obtained! Occasionally a urine specimen is obtained directly from the bladder using a fine needle and syringe (suprapubic aspiration, SPA). This second method has the advantage of providing a specimen that is uncontaminated by any bacteria on the skin, and is quick and safe.

Blood samples are taken because they can provide evidence of infection and, once treatment has begun, can give information on progress. A lumbar puncture may also be performed to obtain a sample of the fluid which surrounds the spinal cord at the lower part of the back (lumbar region). In meningitis changes occur in the composition of the fluid, and the organisms or viruses causing the infection can be identified.

Treatment for infection usually means giving the appropriate antibiotic drugs to combat the problem, but in addition to this some doctors now give components of fresh blood, particularly the white blood cells, whose normal task is to kill bacteria. This may be done by a straightforward infusion of cells, or by an exchange transfusion.

Infection and the digestive system

A few preterm babies develop an inflammation in a section of the wall of their bowel (necrotizing enterocolitis). This causes the abdomen to become distended, and the baby may vomit and pass a little blood in the stool. If there is extensive involvement of the bowel, toxins from invading gut germs may cause serious generalized effects, and occasionally the wall of the bowel may give way (perforate). Peritonitis, which is an inflammation of the lining of the abdominal cavity, results. Some babies may need surgery for the complications of the condition but many, when treated with antibiotics and given adequate nutrition by infusion into a vein, will recover and be able to tolerate milk feeds again.

The brain

The brain is developing in a most dramatic way during the period from 25 weeks' gestation to term. The maturation of brain structures involves the disappearance of some areas which are particularly rich in blood-vessels, and the appearance of many new brain cells. These processes can be disrupted by bleeding (intracranial haemorrhage, intraventricular haemorrhage), or by episodes of oxygen lack (severe hypoxia). The effects will depend on how far the brain has developed and on the extent of the problem. Although most small bleeds have no long term consequences, much of modern newborn care is orientated to preventing these bleeds altogether, and to reducing any periods of low oxygen supply to the brain.

Other investigations

X-rays. Because the various components of body structures absorb X-rays in differing amounts the X-rays that pass through to the sensitive plate behind the tissue being examined provide a pictorial representation of the differing tissue densities. Bones stand out as white, and the lungs, filled with air, appear much darker. X-rays give important information on the size and position of body structures, and on disorders affecting them.

Ultrasound. As with pregnancy, ultrasound has been found to be a particularly useful way of studying the brain, heart, and abdomen, of young babies after birth. It is not yet widely available in neonatal units. Some of the machines have the advantage of being portable so that even a sick baby can be examined without being moved. Ultrasound waves do not pass well through bone and so X-ray investigations are still needed for some examinations.

Computerized Axial X-ray Tomography (CAT scanning) requires bulky, non-portable equipment, so that the baby has to be transported to the scanner. Pictures are built up from the information derived from X-rays passing through tissues under examination, and are displayed as tissue 'slices' or tomograms. This

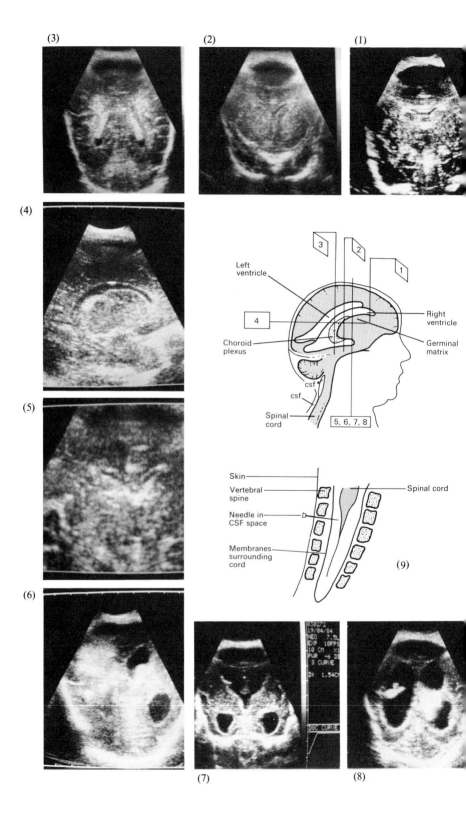

(3)

(2)

(1)

(4)

Left
ventricle

3 2 1

Right
ventricle

4

Choroid
plexus

Germinal
matrix

csf

csf

Spinal
cord

5, 6, 7, 8

(5)

Skin

Vertebral
spine

Spinal cord

Needle in
CSF space

Membranes
surrounding
cord

(9)

(6)

(7)

(8)

technique has been widely used to study the brain, and other internal structures.

Is there a baby in there somewhere?

Amongst the modern high technology of neonatal intensive care allowances for the baby's comfort and need for rest should receive high priority. The humanizing aspects of caring for small babies are easily overlooked by both medical and nursing staff alike. This omission may be a means of self-protection for staff who may feel that they need to shut themselves off from the stressful environment of intensive care. But it can all the more easily arise when the babies being cared for show little in the way of distress no matter what is happening to them. Instead of crying, or protesting, their discomfort may show itself in a less stable blood oxygen level, heart rate, or breathing pattern. Indeed many of the procedures outlined above may disturb the control babies have over these functions.

It is therefore essential that staff and parents try to minimize the discomfort or pain that may arise from some of the procedures that have to be performed. In certain circumstances pain-relieving drugs may be given to help a baby to cope better.

A baby's comfort is reflected in the stability of his breathing pattern and heart rate, in weight gain, in lack of restlessness, and in his wakeful awareness of his surroundings. It can be enhanced by keeping him appropriately warm, and protected from thirst. Some discomforts are avoidable; for example a solvent can be used to remove plasters and sticky tape that hold on monitoring wires and probes, without hurting the baby. Giving a baby a teat or a dummy to suck on, or helping him to suck on his own fingers while painful procedures are carried out may soothe him. The condition

---

Ultrasound pictures of the baby's head reveal the ventricles, which show up black, and brain structures which appear in shades of grey. Coronal views are taken parallel to the forehead (1, 2, 3) and sagittal views are parallel to the side of the head (4). The choroid plexus, which is a cluster of blood vessels from which cerebrospinal fluid (CSF) is produced, appear as white opacities in the normal ventricles.

Haemorrhage in preterm babies can begin in one germinal matrix (5) and may spread into the ventricle as an intraventricular haemorrhage (IVH), (6). The ventricular size can also be measured (7); if excessive accumulation of fluid occurs following a bleed (8) this may be treated by drawing off small amounts via the lumbar spine (9) or directly from the ventricle itself (8).

of preterm babies seems to be more stable when they are nursed on lambswool, are stroked and talked to, and when they are cuddled as soon as they are old enough to tolerate it. All these activities should form part of routine medical and nursing care. (Fig. 5.12)

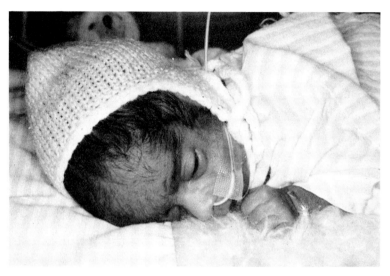

Nursing preterm babies on lambswool seems to lead to a reduction in body movements and better weight gain.

Understaffing, and the associated stresses, can lead to care becoming nothing more than repetitive, automatic, routines. In such circumstances the invasion of a baby's 'privacy' then becomes more overt and obtrusive to the more sensitive staff members, and to the parents. Meeting babies' individual needs, and being alert and responsive to their differing personalities and temperaments, helps to reduce tensions and create a caring, questioning, environment.

Summary

The problems that have been discussed in this chapter may seem to constitute a daunting list, but many can be prevented or resolved. Very rarely would all the procedures described be carried out on any one baby, and some are only required for the treatment and care of very small preterm babies. Many of the problems outlined above do not arise during the first days of life. Rather, it is common for a very preterm baby to pass through periods of needing different kinds of care like ventilatory support, transfusions, oxygen, antibiotics, or phototherapy. It is the very unpredictable nature of a preterm baby's medical condition and progress during the first weeks of life that contributes to parental and staff anxiety, and stress. It can happen that no sooner than one hurdle is apparently overcome than another appears and some babies stay many weeks before going home. Fortunately many preterm babies have few, or even no, medical problems and only need to be in hospital until they are growing well, and feeding normally.

6

The need for
visiting

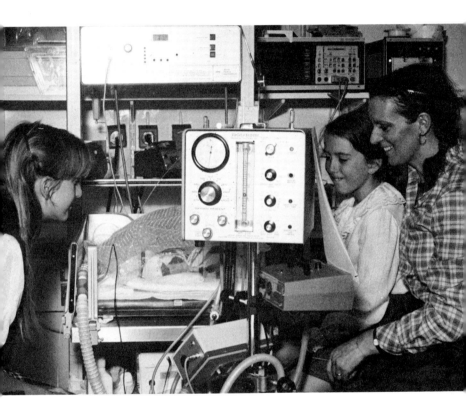

Most units now recognize just how important it is for parents to be encouraged to visit their baby. This change in policy has come about through the increasing awareness that the growth of affection between parents and children is essential to future family harmony. During pregnancy it is normal to imagine how your baby will look and behave. Even though he may be smaller than anticipated, and not yet in perfect health, the first contact is a very emotional moment. Help in coming to terms with the discrepancies between parents' mental images of their baby and the reality enables them to confirm, and accept, their child's uniqueness. If parents are allowed to become involved and to realize how vitally significant they are to the development of this new human being, they will take pride and pleasure as their baby grows and improves in health. Their love and attachment is fostered by interactions with the baby, during which they learn to respond appropriately to his cues, and to recognize how he rewards them by becoming more relaxed and attentive.

Parents need regular contact with their baby if they are to become familiar with his physical, social, and emotional needs, by the time they take him home. It is clear to nurses and parents that each baby has a unique temperament and style of responding which are evident from the earliest days. Parents will find care-giving easier and more satisfying if they are aware of this individuality from the start. Even in the beginning when his condition may be too unstable for him to tolerate being held, parents can do things that contribute to his improved physical well-being; for instance, talking to, and gently stroking him, may soothe and calm a restless baby.

Most parents are anxious about handling their newborn baby; with a preterm infant who appears even more fragile than a full-term baby, these worries are likely to be magnified. By caring for their baby within the supportive environment of the hospital unit, parents develop the confidence and skills that they will need to look after their baby at home.

The first visit

The first visit can be frightening to someone who has never been in a baby unit before. It may be difficult to see the baby in the midst of the many items of equipment, and parents sometimes find the noise of alarms, and the bustle of the staff, rather off-putting. If their baby is in a room where other babies are receiving mechanical breathing support and intensive monitoring, they may feel their baby is in more danger than they had been led to believe. Particularly if they did not not have the opportunity to see him in the delivery room they may be surprised by his appearance, and worried that such a small infant may not survive.

Many units provide an 'instant' photo of the baby soon after admission; this gives parents something to have by them over the next few days, and to show visiting relations. It often becomes a focus for talking about family likeness. Even a photograph is a constant bedside reassurance that, despite his current problems, their baby is 'really there'.

Nursing staff do not expect parents to be competent caretakers on the first visit. They will tell them about the baby's condition, and the equipment which is helping him, and will show them the routines for visits. They may also familiarize them with some of the other staff caring for their baby.

Other visitors to the baby unit

Older children in the family

A few units allow brothers and sisters to visit 'their new baby'. This can be beneficial for children by helping them to become aware of the new arrival, and in preventing distress and anxiety about the baby who hasn't come home. Young children find it difficult to retain an image of the new brother or sister not yet home and benefit by being able to see him or her frequently, and by participating in the caretaking routines. A further advantage of such a policy is that many mothers would not be able to visit as often if they had to make other arrangements for the care of their older children.

However desirable 'sibling visits' may seem to be there is some opposition to them. Young children are often ill with seemingly trivial complaints, but these may be infectious and the child may pass them on before showing any obvious signs of being ill himself. Newborn babies are more vulnerable than older infants so there is always the possibility of infection spreading to other babies in the unit. Because most baby units are very short on space medical staff sometimes feel that active toddlers under foot pose a problem, and

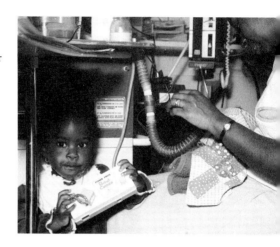

A toddler under foot is little trouble if happily playing near her mother.

that their prying fingers might fiddle with some of the equipment controls. They feel that a mother cannot fully concentrate on caring for her new baby if she is constantly having to monitor the activities of her older children. Some hospitals have solved this latter problem by providing toys on the unit, a 'drop off' playgroup, or even short-term crèche facilities, for visiting children. In others the disadvantages are thought to outweigh the positive benefits, and such visits are not permitted.

Grandparents, other relatives, and friends

Some baby units allow grandparents to visit. Involving them in the baby's care from the beginning reduces the likelihood of the parents being given conflicting advice from an older generation. This involvement of grandparents is especially valuable if they are providing primary support for a single mother. Other relatives and friends are not usually allowed into the unit because of the limited space and nursing workload. However, having a viewing window can enable other visitors to see the baby from an adjacent area.

Procedures for visitors

Handwashing and gowns

In all units visitors will be expected to wash with antibacterial soap before handling the baby. It is important that hands should be dried thoroughly as some germs are transferred more easily from damp skin. It is also advisable to wash *after* changing the baby's nappy to prevent the spread of germs to contact surfaces such as cupboard and door handles.

Some units require visitors to put on a gown or apron to protect their own clothing and theoretically to reduce the transfer of germs to the baby's environment. Others have dispensed with full gowning and masks because research has suggested that most infection is transmitted by hand contact, and therefore scrupulous hand washing and drying are likely to be the best preventive measures against the spread of infections.

Illnesses

If either parent, or anyone else in the family, is unwell—with a cold, viral illness, cough, spots, diarrhoea, or vomiting—it is important to ask the medical staff before going on the unit whether the illness poses any particular risk to the babies there.

Personal belongings and clothing

Visitors should not bring a lot of money or valuable belongings as there may be no safe place to leave them, although they will be given a place to leave coats and outdoor clothing. Neonatal units are kept very warm because small or sick babies have difficulty in regulating their body temperature, and as a consequence visitors find it more comfortable to wear lightweight clothing.

The baby's belongings

Sometimes parents are encouraged to bring in clothing for their baby in order to make the atmosphere more homelike, and they may be asked to wash this clothing at home. However, because of laundering problems, and the risk of belongings being lost or damaged, the majority of units use their own standard newborn night-dresses. Nobody's appearance is improved by being clothed in anonymous plain white hospital clothing stamped 'Hospital Property', and babies are no exception. In some units attempts are being made to remedy this by the provision of more attractive patterned nighties and cot covers. Parents are often encouraged to bring in

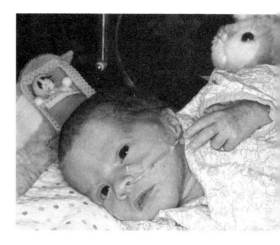

Bright nighties and cot covers make for a more home-like environment and toys provide the baby with something interesting to look at.

a toy, which can be placed at the side of the cot or incubator; this does much to brighten up the environment, as well as giving a baby something to look at as he becomes more alert.

The 'visiting book'

Many units ask parents to keep a record of the time they spend with their baby on each visit, and perhaps to note whether they have been able to hold the baby, or to feed and change him. These records are important as they give staff an indication of which parents are not being given enough opportunity to care for their baby.

At the end of each visit

Parents should be encouraged to talk with the nursing staff before leaving so that alarms can be checked, arrangements for further visiting discussed, and any new information about the baby's progress given.

Making the most of visiting

There can be no hard and fast rules about how often parents should visit their baby, or what they should do during those visits. Both of these will depend on the baby's condition, the baby unit's policies about parental involvement, and the parents' own attitudes, experience, and confidence in handling their baby. Ideally, parents should be able to visit as often and for as long as they wish, gradually increasing the amount and intensity of their contact with the baby so that they are learning a little bit more about him each time. Then by the time he is ready to be taken home they may feel fairly competent and confident in caring for him, being 'in tune' with his needs and personality. Because there are different priorities for parental involvement immediately after birth, compared with when the baby is older, these periods will be discussed separately.

The early days: the growth of love and affection

Some preterm infants, particularly those of more than 34 weeks gestation, may have an easy birth, experience no respiratory problems, and be stable enough to be cared for by their parents on the first day or so. The majority of those of earlier gestation, however, are monitored in the warmth of an incubator, and may require respiratory support, with the result that their parents will not be able to hold them for long periods. A few infants find it so difficult to control their temperature, heart-rate, or breathing at the beginning, that 'minimal handling' will be advised. In this situation the parents' role may be limited to watching and talking to their baby.

The natural reaction after a birth is for parents to want to hold, touch, and caress their new infant, and they are bound to be disappointed if their infant's condition prevents this. To gaze longingly and lovingly at him through the side of an incubator is not the same thing at all. For parents whose access to their baby remains limited, a series of photographs, in addition to those given them on admission of their baby, is greatly cherished. Sometimes parents long to see their baby's face behind the face mask, and if told of this desire staff may offer to take a photograph when the mask is changed since the parents may not be around at that time.

Normally one of the earliest tasks of parenthood is learning how to soothe and comfort a baby, and protect him from hurt and discomfort. When the baby is isolated in an incubator, and is exposed to painful medical procedures, most parents feel helpless to provide such caring. They hesitate to ask doctors to be more gentle in taking blood samples, or in chiding nurses who brusquely handle their baby for weighing or changing. Sometimes they are told by the medical staff that 'newborn infants don't feel pain', and thus are made to feel even more unreasonable in asking anyone to alter their practices. In fact parents can do a great deal to make procedures less traumatic for their baby and to give him opportunities to associate touch with comfort, instead of with pain. They may be permitted to stroke the baby's body, or to let him suck on their finger, as a distraction during an uncomfortable procedure. If the baby is able to come out of the incubator, then he can be held snuggly against his mother's body, or swaddled in a sheet to comfort him, while a blood sample is being taken.

Talking to or singing to the baby are ways to add comforting sounds to any handling procedures. Parents are often acutely aware of the isolation of their baby in an incubator, and feel that the perspex is a barrier preventing interaction with him, particularly talking. However it is often possible for monitor bleep volumes to be turned down to enable the baby to hear his parent's voice, or a soft rattle, or music box. Many parents therefore see the progression from an open overhead heated platform to the confines of an incubator as a retrograde step, rather than the promotion it represents in medical terms. Staff should encourage parents to reach in and touch their baby and, if possible, should take the baby out for brief periods on the parent's lap, even if he is still connected to monitors and needing supplementary oxygen.

The baby who is seriously ill

Some parents, and professionals too, have questioned the desirability of a family becoming too close to a baby whose condition is serious. Parents may deliberately distance themselves from the baby to avoid becoming attached to him. They feel that frequent or prolonged visiting will lead to feelings of love and affection that will later prove too painful should the baby not survive.

However there are many reasons why it is important to discourage this attitude. Most parents overestimate the severity of their baby's condition, often believing that he will die when there are in fact few medical concerns about him. Although some small preterm infants have severe respiratory problems in the early days, most make a rapid recovery. Continuing advances in the monitoring and treatment of such babies make doctors increasingly optimistic about the outcome, even of some of the smallest infants. Interviews

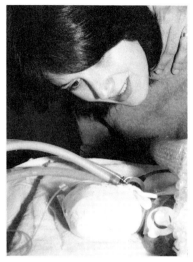
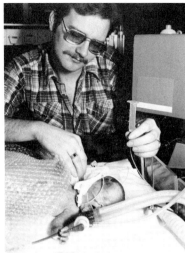

Even ill babies, like these two of 26 weeks' gestation, can be talked to, stroked, and tube-fed by their parents.

with parents suggest that when the baby does survive it is more difficult to come to love and accept him if they had initially avoided much involvement. When the infant has died parents usually regret not having visited more often. They find it difficult to summon up a memory of him as a real person, and thus hold no special image that they can later cherish. They may feel guilty that they did not offer him as much affection during the short time he was with them as they would have done had he been healthy.

Of course every parent responds differently to their own baby's condition, but in general it is advantageous for them to be optimistic about the baby's outlook, and to visit him as much as possible. Giving him a name and, in accordance with religious beliefs, baptizing him, will help to ensure that he assumes a special identity. Stroking and talking to him, even if he seems too small or too ill to benefit, helps parents to feel that they have done the most for him that is possible.

As the baby gets bigger

As the baby's condition improves the parents will begin to assume more of the caretaking tasks when they come to visit. Some keep a diary of their baby's progress and derive pleasure from it in the years to come. An example may be found at the end of this chapter (p. 79). It is quite common for parents to feel some trepidation at being 'left in charge' when changing a nappy or giving a tube-feed for the first time. Nurses are not always aware of how much anxiety is caused by their leaving the room at that moment, or by putting too much pressure on parents to carry out caretaking tasks when they are not wholly confident. If the atmosphere in the unit is conducive to parents asking for help then they will do so. If they are treated like patients, or if they are regarded as impediments to the baby's care, they may well be too inhibited to ask for assistance, or too frightened to try again. Mothers are often particularly anxious about bathing their baby when they go home because they have usually not had very many opportunities to do so beforehand. The staff can help by being aware of such concerns, and by arranging for the baby to have more frequent baths in the week or so preceding discharge.

As the baby grows he will also become more alert and attentive to his surroundings, and the visits will become more rewarding. It is important for him to learn to associate feeding time with being held and cuddled and talked to, and to come to learn that his signs of hunger are recognized and answered. The nurses do not always have the time to talk to and play with a baby during and after a feed, and they may not be able to immediately pick up a baby who is crying. This is why parents have a major responsibility to help their baby to expect to be cared for when he cries, and to learn to recognize the familiar voices and faces of his regular caretakers. Even babies who are being tube-fed should be held and talked to rather than left in their cots. As they progress to a less frequent feeding schedule it is important for them to be wakened so that they can come to associate wakefulness with feeding and being talked to.

The nurses may have noted that a particular baby is usually more awake at one time of day rather than another, and so they may recommend parents to visit at that time. Suggestions for ways of increasing alertness in the baby when feeding him are considered in more detail in Chapter 7, and in relation to promoting optimal development, in Chapter 8. A mother should be encouraged to stay for a whole feed–sleep cycle on some occasions in order to learn how her baby wakes for a feed, and how he settles back to sleep afterwards, if indeed he does! Much of the time may be spent with her baby asleep and she should feel free just to read, knit, or talk, by the side of his cot.

Practical problems in visiting the baby

The early days

During the week following the birth most mothers have times when they feel sore and weak. Following complications, such as bleeding or hypertension, they may be advised to stay in bed, or may even be connected to 'drips' which makes walking around impossible. These problems make it difficult for mothers to visit as often as they would like. They may feel guilty about not doing enough for their baby, and often at the same time resentful that the medical staff don't make it easier for them to have contact with their baby. The few hospitals which provide 'rooming-in' facilities for preterm infants and their mothers set an example in this respect. Some postnatal wards are very supportive in this situation and regularly take the mother in a wheelchair to visit her baby, or bring the baby to her for short periods in a 'transport incubator'. But in most cases the mother will have to rely on photographs of her baby and reports from her partner about the baby's condition until she is able to go herself. The paediatricians attending babies on the postnatal wards may be the most appropriate people to liaise with the baby unit, and so ensure that the mother is given accurate information about the baby's progress and that her questions and anxieties are fully addressed.

When the baby is in another hospital

When mother and baby are in separate hospitals it is important for her partner to visit the baby, and to keep in regular touch with the baby unit. The mother may not have ready access to a telephone and so will be unable to talk to the doctors there directly. Again the liaison role of the paediatric and nursing staff on her postnatal ward is crucial in imparting up-to-date medical information about the baby. Once the mother is more mobile arrangements may be made for her to be taken by hospital transport, or ambulance, to visit her baby.

Medical staff need to be aware of the distress of the mother

whose baby is miles away in another hospital as feelings of help-
lessness, remoteness, and depression, are exacerbated in this situation. With many different people involved in the care of mother
and baby it is not unusual for parents to receive conflicting reports
about their baby which only serve to heighten their anxiety, and
make them distrustful of the medical personnel. If the mother has
no post-partum medical problems she may prefer to be discharged
early from hospital so that she can maximize the time available to
see her baby.

The dilemma of remaining in hospital or returning home

Some mothers find it unbearably distressing to remain in the postnatal ward while their baby is some distance away in the baby unit;
they prefer to go home as early as possible and visit frequently.
This may be the most satisfactory solution, particularly if there are
other young children at home. Mothers who choose to do so must
not be made to feel as if they are 'abandoning' their baby, or are
any less concerned about him than mothers who remain in hospital.

Some mothers might need to stay in hospital because of an
operative delivery, or postnatal complications. Others might choose
to remain so that they can be near the baby continually, or at least
until they have reassured themselves that he is 'out of danger'. If
a mother is breast-feeding, and her baby is likely to remain in the
baby unit for only a few weeks, the staff may arrange for her to be
on the postnatal ward until the two of them can be discharged
home together. Similarly, if regular visiting is impractical because
of distance—particularly true in the case of regional referral
centres—it may sometimes be possible to arrange long-stay facilities for the mother. Alternatively, once the baby no longer requires
intensive care he may be transferred back to a unit that is nearer
to the parents' home.

It is important to recognize that, quite apart from the stress of
worrying about her baby's condition, the institutional nature of
hospital itself can upset a mother. The 'long-stay' mother faces the
loss of privacy, the monotony of hospital food, and of inflexible
routines, 'bossy' nurses and medical staff who may treat her as a
patient rather than a parent, and the sheer boredom of the long
days. Not surprisingly increased tearfulness and depressive symptoms are therefore quite common. Inevitably the mother will feel

guilty about leaving her husband or partner to cope on his own, and miss the physical intimacy, tenderness, and sharing of feelings, which are not easily expressed during his visits to the hospital.

Financial worries

It is easy to underestimate the cost of travelling to and from the hospital, even when it is only a short distance. If a child-minder is being employed for other children in the family the expenditure may seem never-ending. These problems can sometimes be helped with advice from the unit's social worker, and the hospital may provide tokens for the mother's meals.

Conflicting demands

It may be difficult to find the right balance between the needs of the mother and family and those which the medical and nursing staff regard as ideal when it comes to visiting and caring for the new baby. It is not uncommon for parents to find unrealistic demands placed on them. Parents need to be given ample opportunity to discuss with the nursing staff how they can best use the time to learn about their baby's needs, without neglecting family responsibilities.

The mother's needs

With everyone's attention focused on the baby it is easy to forget the mother's needs at this time. In the first few days she will still require considerable rest. Over the weeks that she comes to visit the baby it is important for her not to neglect regular meals and extra rest periods since the fatigue of travelling to and from the baby unit, and the associated emotional stress, can be considerable. If the mother is providing breast-milk, it is particularly important for her to be aware that she should have an extra 500 calories or so per day in the form of meat, vegetables, and dairy products, to maintain a good milk supply. Many hospitals give meal tokens for mothers visiting their children in hospital, which in theory ensures that they do not have to skimp on a midday meal.

Once the mother has gone home without her baby people may be quick to assume that she 'has it easy'—no nappies to wash, no broken nights. This attitude ignores the heartache caused by separation, and underestimates the amount of time spent travelling. The effect on physical and mental health of worry about the baby, and guilt about not fulfilling everyone's expectations, may pass unrecognised.

The father's needs

While the mother is in hospital the father will have many additional responsibilities such as preparing his own meals, caring for their home, and answering endless enquiries about the baby from friends and relatives. Sometimes the medical staff are unaware that a father who comes in to visit his baby might have skipped breakfast because there's no one to eat it with; he may have done a full day's work, spent a tiring journey by public transport, or in a traffic jam, and then skipped the evening meal as well in order to spend time at the hospital. If the nurses then inadvertently imply that he is not visiting often enough he may feel even more of a failure. The cultural stereotype of the 'strong silent' male means that many fathers cannot openly show their intense worry or disappointment to others, and may wish to avoid adding to their partner's distress by appearing not to be 'in control'.

Needs of other children in the family

Other children in the family will not fully appreciate what is going on with the baby, or why he requies so much attention from their parents. Suggestions for dealing with the older children's anxieties, expectations, and changes in behaviour, are dealt with more fully in Chapter 10. However, when discussing times for parental visits some consideration should be given to their needs. Young children are very dependent on home routines such as set mealtimes, daily outings, or particular stories being read before bed. If at all possible visits to the new baby should be planned so as not to disrupt such activities, or at least not to do so on a regular basis.

Practical solutions

It is rarely possible to please everyone, but many problems of visiting can be tackled successfully with co-operation between staff

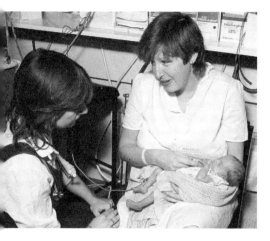

Regular talks with the doctors and nurses enable concerns to be voiced and answered, and ensure that parents are closely involved with all that is happening to their baby.

and parents. If parents find that the baby's feeding times conflict with set family routines then the nursing staff may be able to re-schedule feeds, and will be glad to have had the problem brought to their attention. Parents should play their part in reducing staff inconvenience and annoyance by notifying the nurses when they are unable to make a particular visit so that the baby is not left waiting unnecessarily for a feed, bath, or cuddle.

Although the medical staff often appear busy, they would much prefer parents to ask them questions directly than to go away confused about their baby's condition. It may take considerable courage to ask the doctor to go over things several times, but he or she should understand that it takes a while for non-medical people to grasp the facts about a particular condition or treatment. A genuine desire to know the details about their baby's care should be seen as a positive attribute, rather than a time-consuming incon-venience.

Diary of the parents of a 31-week baby

Week 1

d. 1   Talked to her. Took photos.

d. 3   Talked (morning). Talked (afternoon). She opened her eyes (evening).

d. 7   Talked. Heard Donna cry for the first time.

Week 2

d. 9   Held our Donna for the first time and had photos taken as well!

d. 10 Held her for a long cuddle (morning). We both held her again (evening).

d. 12 The boys held Donna today.

d. 13 Changed her nappy for the first time today.

Week 3

d. 15 Sat her up to bring up wind.

d. 16 Held Donna and she smiled!

d. 18 Donna was wide awake this morning.

d. 19 Took photos. Dad held her and tube fed her.

d. 21 Very pleased with her progress and enjoy giving her a cuddle.

Week 4

d. 22 When we came in we were surprised to find our girl in the next room (cold nursery).

d. 27 Pulled my usual faces at her. She looks beautiful!

d. 28 Donna looked so comfy that I didn't want to disturb her.

Week 5

d. 29 Very surprised at her size now. Incubator doors open today!

d. 30 So surprised to see Donna in her cot already! Took some photos.

d. 34 Today I just watched the sister (bottle) feed Little Wonder.

d. 35 Donna was *very* well-behaved tonight.

Week 6

d. 36 Stayed all day with Donna. Fed her with a bottle for the first time! Mum thinks her Donna is FAB! She is much more like a baby what with her bottle-feed.

d. 40 Donna made sure I (Dad) had a hard time when I changed her— my first *solo* change. She must have been worried over me doing it for her.

d. 42 I (Mum) arrived at the wrong time for Donna's feed time but we enjoyed a lovely cuddle.

Week 7

d. 43 Today we had a long time together. She seems a very placid baby. I think both Ann and myself are just the same.

d. 45 Donna made me (Dad) change her twice tonight. Still, it's all very good practice for me.

d. 46 We're told super-girl comes home next Wednesday. Please God.

7

Nutrition and feeding

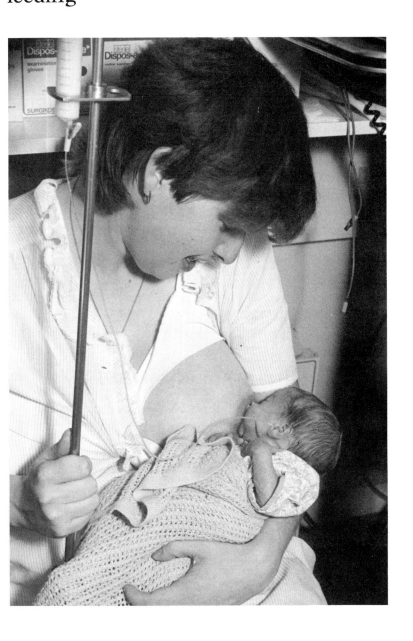

Nutrition and digestion

At birth, both the preterm and the small-for-gestational-age baby have little in the way of energy reserves. Yet they have high energy requirements. In the past, because early feeds are often vomited, or cause apnoeic episodes, it was customary not to feed these babies for several days. Recognition of early nutritional needs has radically altered this attitude to early 'feeding'.

Energy requirements

All young infants need nourishment for growth and muscle activity. Nutritional sources provide the energy for all body processes, and energy requirements are particularly high in the preterm infant, whether well or sick. The exact amounts of nutrients, electrolytes, minerals, vitamins, and water to be given, are calculated on the basis of a baby's weight, gestation, and on results from blood and urine tests.

The problems of providing adequate quantities of nutrients

In the past it was observed that these small babies seemed to have insufficient energy for breast- or bottle-feeding; as mentioned above, they frequently had apnoeic episodes during feeds, sometimes with regurgitation and posseting (spitting up) of milk.

There are many reasons for this apparent inability to cope with normal feeding. Sucking itself is particularly weak before about 32 weeks' gestation. Co-ordination of sucking and swallowing is not achieved much before 34 weeks. The stomach itself is very small, and the passage of milk from it is slow. The valve-like mechanism at the entry to the stomach which keeps milk down, preventing it from passing back up into the throat and mouth, functions poorly. Regurgitation of milk is therefore frequent, and if the milk is inhaled from the throat a baby's breathing is likely to be affected. Normally this 'valve' relaxes during 'burping' to allow 'wind' to escape, but otherwise remains closed until the milk has passed through. Filling the stomach of a baby who is lying flat pushes up on the main muscle of breathing, the diaphragm, and it is now recognised that this can reduce breathing movements and cause a fall in the oxygen level in the baby's blood; a fall in oxygen level may precipitate apnoea. Small amounts of milk given frequently, which do not distend the stomach, are therefore better tolerated than larger feeds given every three or four hours.

The hormones involved in promoting the muscular propulsion of food through the digestive tract are not released in a normal, co-ordinated way, in preterm babies. Muscular contractions of the intestinal wall serve to mix the milk with digestive enzymes, and with other compounds which make the milk fats easier to digest. Only in a suitably digested form can nutrients be absorbed by passing through the lining cells of the digestive tract. The release of enzymes and the other factors important for digestion is reduced in the preterm infant so that nutrients are wasted, being passed unabsorbed in the baby's stools.

Slow transit of milk through the intestine, together with poor absorption, and a lot of gas formation, often gives rise to a full-looking tummy. This prominence, or 'distension', may result in loops of the digestive system being easily visible through the thin skin of the preterm baby's abdomen. Food wastage in stools can result in inadequate amounts of nutrients being available for growth.

How nutrition is provided

Part of the early energy requirements are now met by giving solutions of glucose intravenously. However glucose is only one of the baby's needs. Amino-acids are the basic units from which body proteins are made, and sources of fat, vitamins, and minerals, are also essential. When babies are ill, or are having difficulty absorbing enough nutrients from milk, their needs can now be met with more complex intravenous formulations—so-called intravenous or total parenteral nutrition. These are specially prepared to contain all essential components.

To reduce the work that babies have to put into feeding, and to provide nutrition for those too immature to suck, feeds are given by tube (gavage feeding). Soft, fine, tubes are used, and are passed from the nose to the stomach (nasogastric), or through the mouth (orogastric), and are held in place by a piece of sticky tape. Special tubes can also be passed beyond the stomach into the jejunum (naso-jejunal).

The position of the gastric tube is checked before each feed.

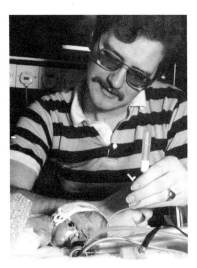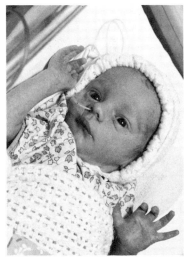

A tube passed through the nose is used for feeding babies who are either too ill or too immature to suck and swallow for themselves. The sooner parents can be involved with this activity, the more confidence and pride they feel.

Gentle suction (aspiration) may be applied to the tube before each feed to check that all the milk from the previous feed has passed on from the stomach to the small intestine where absorption takes place. Should regurgitation of feeds be a problem then the volume given may have to be reduced and made good by increasing the intravenous intake, or the decision may be made to site a tube in the jejunum.

Jejunal placement introduces the milk beyond the stomach. Sometimes stomach fluids are continuously aspirated, using a second tube passed through the mouth; this minimizes the chance of regurgitation and inhalation of any fluid from the stomach into the lungs. The aspirated fluid (gastric aspirate) can be passed back down the jejunal tube so that important constituents are not lost. The absence of a cough or gag (choking) reflex before about 32 weeks' gestation means that a baby born before this time is at risk from inhaling regurgitated feeds. This risk is further reduced by lying the baby on his tummy after feeds, or by having him on his side, so that any regurgitated milk dribbles out of his mouth rather than passing into his windpipe. Regurgitation is less likely if the baby is left undisturbed after a feed.

Continuous aspiration of stomach contents is also carried out whenever there is evidence of an obstruction to the passage of food through the digestive system. When such an obstruction is present it is usual to find green bile in the fluid that has been aspirated. Bile may also flow back into the stomach from the small intestine during jejunal feeding because the soft tube that is used interferes with closure of the outlet at the lower end of the stomach.

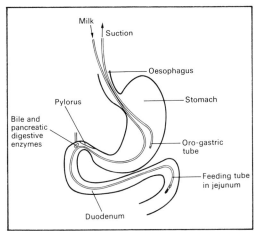

In transpyloric feeding, the tube is passed beyond the outlet from the stomach (the pylorus) into the duodenum or jejunum. A second tube in the stomach may be used to aspirate the stomach secretions and so reduce the chance of regurgitation and inhalation into the lungs.

Weight gain and growth

It might be reasonably supposed that the dramatic rate of growth which had been present before birth would continue unabated afterwards. However, not only does the newborn baby have to expend energy on keeping warm, on breathing, and on a whole range of activities that were not needed before birth, much food energy is wasted, as discussed above. In the past many small pre-term babies did not regain their birthweights for four or five weeks—a period of relative 'starvation'. Although on current feeding regimes many regain their birthweight by two or three weeks, compared with the seven to ten days in most full-term babies, there are many ups and downs in weight gain. Weight losses frequently accompany minor set backs or illnesses and are the rule in the first few days of life.

The documentation of weight gain or loss is an important indicator of health and nutritional requirements, and of whether these needs are being met. Knowledge of a baby's weight forms the basis for calculations of fluid volumes, nutrients, and mineral requirements, as well as drug and antibiotic dosages. Intakes are often adjusted on the basis of the appearance of the baby, and on blood test results. Continued weight loss requires investigation and appropriate treatment.

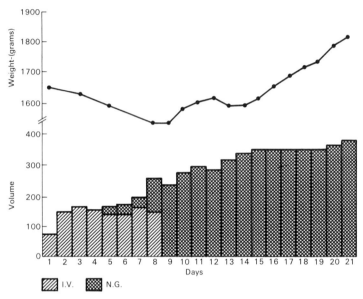

Many preterm babies, after an initial loss of body water, regain their birth weight by 2 to 3 weeks; fluctuations in the rate of weight gain are common and often accompany any later illnesses. The chart illustrates the daily intake of a 30-week gestation baby and her weight record. 'I.V.' indicates volume of intravenous fluid given; 'N.G.' represents the volume of milk given naso-gastrically.

Vitamin and iron deficiencies

When born early babies 'miss out' on the period during which they build up their stores of iron and vitamins. These are mainly acquired from their mothers during the last two months of the pregnancy. Supplements of vitamins A, D, E, K, and folic acid may be needed to meet the demands of a rapidly growing baby, and extra iron may be needed in addition to that present in breast or formula milks.

Bone development

Calcium, phosphorus, vitamin D, and certain hormones, are essential for the normal deposition of minerals (mineralization) in the protein substructure of bone. When preterm babies start to grow rapidly the lengthening of bones may outstrip the rate of mineralization—especially if any of the above components is deficient. Bones of the head are soft and deformable, which explains the head flattening that can occur in the early weeks of a preterm baby's life. Softness and flexibility of the bones of the rib cage cause breathing difficulties and the in-drawing of the chest wall that is seen. This chest recession is frequently observed during any respiratory distress in the newborn period. Ensuring an adequate intake of minerals and vitamin D may help prevent later defects of bone mineralization—known as rickets. Blood tests and X-rays may reveal this disorder, in which case appropriate treatment is begun.

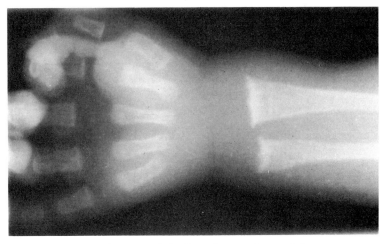

This X-ray of a wrist of a preterm baby shows the ragged, expanded appearance of the growing ends of the long bones of the forearm due to defective bone mineralization (rickets).

Which milk is best?

The baby's mother's own expressed breast-milk is well digested by most preterm infants. The living cells and antibodies in human milk are not present in artificial formulas. They help to minimize the growth of bacteria in the baby's digestive system, reducing the chance of gastroenteritis, and perhaps of necrotizing enterocolitis. The active enzymes—which are destroyed in the preparation of artificial formulas, and to a lesser extent by pasteurization of breast-milk—aid digestion, so that the proportion of nutrients absorbed is increased. Because the protein in breast-milk is 'human' not cow, goat, or soy protein, the chance of the baby becoming allergic ('sensitized') to the milk is minimal.

To ensure its safety, donor milk is heated (pasteurized) and then frozen and stored in the hospital's milk bank until required.

For the extremely immature preterm baby even breast-milk may not have enough protein, salts or minerals. This is in spite of the greater amount of protein that is present in the milk of the mothers of these babies. Supplements can be given whenever the milk is judged to be insufficient. Similarly, normal formula feeds may not provide enough nutrients for these particular babies. Nowadays some new artificial milks are specially manufactured for very immature babies; they contain what are considered to be optimal amounts of all the necessary ingredients for these infants. However it is doubtful whether such formulas will surpass the excellence of breast-milk from the baby's own mother, provided excessive heating of her milk has not occurred, and that supplements are added when needed.

Some hospitals utilize breast-milk from other lactating mothers to reduce babies' exposure to cows' milk based formulas. This milk may be expressed after a mother has fed her own baby, or collected as 'drip' breast-milk as it spontaneously comes from the breast when her baby is nursing on the other side.

Breast-milk and the establishment of breast-feeding

Many people are surprised by the appearance of breast-milk. It is naturally slightly blue in colour, and has an apparently 'thin' consistency. When compared with cows milk this can lead mothers who have not breast-fed before to assume that their milk is not adequate for feeding their baby. The appearance, consistency, and quantity, may differ within a feed, and from feed to feed, but over the day a baby will receive the right balance of vitamins, minerals, fats, and carbohydrates, suitable for him. Colostrum, the fluid produced by the breasts in the few days after the baby's birth, is almost clear or yellowish. This has a slightly different composition from the 'true' milk which comes in afterwards, and contains more minerals, protein and vitamin A, and rather less fat and sugar. Colostrum is easy to digest and transfers important immunities from the mother to the baby. Colostrum and milk are produced together for about a fortnight, which may account for the variety of colours and consistencies of milk seen over this time.

During a breast-feed the baby gets his milk *not* by sucking on the nipple but by pressing his gums on the milk sacs behind the areola. To accomplish this manoeuvre it has been pointed out that a full-term newborn baby has jaw muscles which are, relatively, three times more powerful than those of an adult. When he sucks, the nipple is drawn well back on to his tongue creating a vacuum seal that allows him to 'rest' without coming off the breast.

A small quantity of milk (foremilk) is immediately available when the baby starts to feed. However the stimulation of sucking sets off the release of a chain of hormones in the mother, including oxytocin. This, after some seconds or minutes, causes the involuntary 'let-down' reflex in the breast during which the walls of the

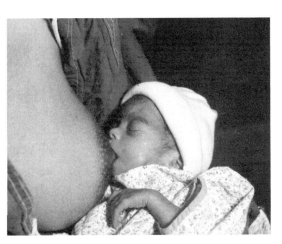

Close contact and careful positioning of the baby's head are necessary to ensure that she draws the areola well into her mouth and that her nose remains unobstructed during sucking, swallowing, and breathing.

milk sacs contract and release the rest of the milk (hind-milk). At this point a baby often has little sucking to do, and may indeed cough and splutter as he tries to cope with the milk flow.

The let-down reflex may be experienced as a warm, tingly sensation in the breast, milk dripping from one or both breasts, and, in the early days, cramps in the uterus produced as its muscular walls contract under the influence of the oxytocin. Other women are unaware of the reflex but as long as milk is released there is no need to become concerned. It is not unusual, early on, to find that this reflex works when just thinking about the baby, or as a mother is preparing to breast-feed.

Supply and demand

Breast-feeding (lactation) works on a supply and demand system—the *more* frequently the baby sucks—or the milk is expressed—the *more* milk will be produced. A newborn baby would normally suckle at least six, and usually more, times a day; some full-term babies demand a feed every 2–3 hours. Because breast-milk is so easily digested it passes through the digestive system quite quickly, and thus a breast-fed baby may feel 'hungry' more often than a baby on cows milk formula.

In order to begin producing a good milk flow the mother of a preterm baby needs to mimic the frequent suckling of a full-term baby by expressing milk regularly. If possible she should begin by expressing every *2–3* hours, and then adjust the 'supply' to meet the 'demand'. Every four hours should be the maximum interval in the early days or it may be difficult to get the milk flowing. However, many mothers find they can get away with not expressing in the middle of the night, and it is true that if you are too tired then your milk supply can diminish. Often mothers find that their breasts become engorged (swollen and hard) in the night after 6–8 hours, or that they cannot express as much milk after leaving out night pumpings. Each individual needs to find out what suits her. The most essential fact to remember is *if* your milk flow seems to be decreasing *express more often*.

A small baby will only need 100 ml or so per kg body weight ($1\frac{1}{2}$ oz per lb) in the first few days, so this is the sort of volume to be aiming for. By the end of the first week he may be taking 150 ml per kg, in which case you will be trying to express more.

Expressing milk

If a baby is not yet able to feed directly from the breast then it will be necessary to 'express' milk, which can then be given to him by tube, or stored until he is ready for it. There are two ways of expressing, either by hand, or by using one of the many different pumps that are available. It is important to remember that each mother might find a different method of expressing to be best for her— depending on the shape of her breasts, the degree of engorgement she feels, and the tenderness of her nipples. At the very beginning of lactation, or after a very premature delivery, some mothers may need the controlled, even pressure of an electric pump, but switch comfortably to a hand pump later on, or to using manual expression just to relieve fullness before the baby begins to feed. The following sections briefly summarize the methods of expressing using the different pumping systems. Most neonatal units or maternity wards have some nursing or midwifery staff who are experienced in helping mothers of preterm infants express their milk. Breast-feeding support groups and counsellors from the community can offer advice, put mothers in touch with experienced breast-feeders, and loan out breast pumps (see Appendix 2, p. 232).

Hand expressing

First, holding the whole breast in both hands, exert pressure all round the breast by moving your fingers down toward the areola. Then squeeze the milk sacs behind the areola gently until the milk comes out. Rotate your hand around the breast to empty all the sacs, being careful not to let it 'slide' on the skin as this can cause chafing.

Hand expression takes practice and is learnt most easily by watching someone else. Some mothers find it a slow and tedious way of producing enough milk for a preterm baby but it is an invaluable technique to learn for relieving the pressure on an engorged breast; it is also useful for expressing a little milk at the beginning of a feed so that the baby is not swamped by the initial rush of milk.

Bulb pumps

The most common and inexpensive pump has a flanged cone-shaped tube with a bulb on one end. After wetting the inside of

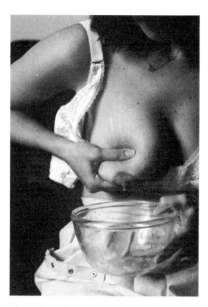

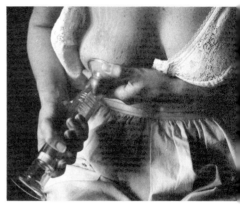

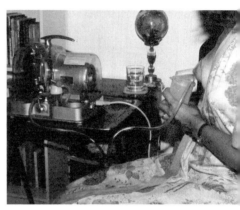

A mother's breast milk can be expressed and given to her baby. Three methods are illustrated: expression by hand, by hand-operating plunger (piston) pump, and by using an electric suction pump.

the cone, or the breast, squeeze the bulb slightly before placing it on the breast. Continue squeezing the bulb to milk the breast. While some mothers are happy with this type of pump others find it the least satisfactory of the hand pumps because it may make nipples and breasts sore.

Plunger pumps

These pumps work on a piston principle and usually convert to a feeding bottle. A plastic 'cup' is placed over the breast and held firmly with one hand. The other hand is used with a push-pull motion on the outer syringe which draws out the milk. Once a milk supply has been established and you get the 'knack' of it it is possible to express 80–100 ml almost as quickly as with an electric pump. Different sized adaptors are usually available for the nipple end of the syringe, and a good fit (and hence suction) can make a lot of difference to how well it works.

Electric pumps

The principle of electric pumps is to apply an intermittent suction to the breast. A glass cup is placed over the breast with the nipple well centred and as suction is applied from the pump milk flows into the collecting bottle beneath the cup. The pump is used with the cup applied to each breast for a few minutes. Depending on the pump design, certain of the components, such as the cup, bottle, bottle-stopper, and tubing, need sterilization between sessions.

Hand-operated pumps can be borrowed or purchased relatively cheaply. Electric pumps are often available from midwifery departments, neonatal units, or from breast-feeding support groups.

Many mothers of tiny babies find it frustrating and disappointing to express milk for many weeks without the emotional and physical satisfaction of having their baby on the breast. Sometimes mothers describe expressing as being 'very distant' from real breast-feeding, while others are completely put off by the mechanical nature of electric pumps. Having to express their milk with little privacy on a neonatal unit can seem 'unnatural' or 'disgusting', even to mothers who would have no qualms about nursing their baby in public.

If there are suddenly increased concerns over her baby, or if there are problems at home, then it is usual for mothers to find that their milk supply decreases. It is still worth persevering with expressing, for once the anxiety has passed you should find that your milk production will get back to normal.

Expressing for your baby gives him all the advantages of your breast milk and in time both of you will come to enjoy the comfort and emotional satisfaction of breast-feeding.

Collecting and storing breast milk

The following section sets out general guidelines for handling breast milk. Individual units vary in their instructions about containers and procedures, so always consult one of the nursing staff caring for your baby first.

It is essential that your hands are scrupulously clean, but it is not necessary to wash your nipples. The equipment used for expressing—bottles, other containers, pump parts—must be sterile. If the hospital does not supply these in sealed packs it will be necessary to scrub them clean with a brush and then sterilize them by one of the following methods:

(1) soaking in a cold water sterilizing system (using tablets or liquid as directed), for a minimum of 30 minutes, or as specified on the packet;

(2) bringing to boiling point and then simmering for a further 15 minutes;

(3) running through a dishwasher on a cycle which reaches 180 °F/90 °C.

Plastic or pyrex containers should be used for freezing milk since 'disposable' bottle liners can leach out chemicals into the milk when frozen.

Expressed milk can be stored safely in a refrigerator for 24 hours, or alternatively it can be frozen immediately and brought into the hospital in a 'cool' bag, or packed with 'ice packs'. Each sample is better put into a *separate* bottle and clearly labelled with your baby's name, and the date and time that it was expressed, since only small quantities may be needed for any one feed. Once the baby is home and milk is being expressed to save for the occasional bottle-feed or 'top-up', then it can be put into a single bottle. In that case the bottle should be well shaken to mix-up the layers when defrosted.

Successful breast-feeding

Because of the early delivery, anxieties about the baby, and the added problems of travelling, and general fatigue, it may seem quite difficult to establish breast-feeding. However a number of common problems are easier to cope with if you know their causes.

Engorged breasts

Engorgement refers to breasts which become tense and hard, sometimes with swelling of the areola. Many mothers experience a brief period of engorgement when their milk first comes in, but this usually lasts no more than a few days. However mothers of preterm babies may find that engorgement is more of a problem since they may not be regularly pumping their breasts, or their baby is sleepy and not very efficient at emptying the breasts at each feed time.

Sore breasts can be painful, and it is so easy at this point to feel like giving up the idea of breast-feeding altogether. If you can remember that the condition is likely to be short-lived and that there are ways to make it tolerable then it will probably pass before you have lost all your confidence. The following are helpful points:

1. Express more frequently, but for shorter periods. If the baby is already suckling then feed him 'little and often'.
2. Make certain that each breast is completely emptied of milk. If the baby does not drink it all then express the rest.
3. Massage the breasts, particularly the lumpy areas, while feeding or expressing.
4. Both warmth and cold can soothe the discomfort. Try an ice pack, or a hot water bottle, or heating pad.

Very occasionally an abscess (infection) can begin to develop. Any redness of the breast, fever, or persistent engorgement, should be checked by a nurse, midwife, or doctor.

Sore nipples

Tenderness of the nipples is common at the beginning of breast-feeding. Mothers who are expressing occasionally find that the pumps chafe at the skin so it is important to use a flange that fits firmly, but comfortably, on the areola (as the baby would be) and not to draw the nipple too vigorously into the pump. Soreness is often caused by the baby being poorly positioned on the breast so that he 'drags down' on the nipple rather than taking the surrounding areola into his mouth. As your baby may still be quite small when you begin to put him to the breast it may help to place him on several pillows in your lap to bring him up to a comfortable height. When taking your baby off the breast be careful to break the suction by putting your finger in the corner of his mouth. Just pulling him off is likely to make your nipples sore.

Insufficient milk

A few mothers of preterm infants fail to establish an adequate milk supply, particularly if the baby was born before 30 weeks' gestation. This may be because their system is not ready to produce milk so early in the pregnancy, but it is more likely to be a combination of factors such as infrequent expressing, poor 'technique', worry, and exhaustion.

Mothers who have successfully breast-fed their preterm infants have found the following suggestions helpful:

1. Try to relax and look forward to the time when your baby will be feeding normally. Thinking about him and looking at his photograph may do the trick.
2. Warmth also stimulates milk production; warm flannels applied several times a day before expressing can help, while some mothers prefer to express while sitting in a hot bath!
3. Producing milk uses up calories (at least 500 *extra* calories per day), and often makes mothers thirsty. A snack and drink just before, or during expressing or nursing, often seems to increase milk flow.
4. When trying to pump milk in the over-hot environment of the neonatal unit it is especially important to have a cool drink to hand. Beer and wine, which help relaxation, have long been recommended, in small quantities, as tonics for the breast-feeding mother.
5. When a baby feeds he nuzzles against the breast and tongues the nipple and areola, providing a distinctive kind of stimulation. Using clean hands try to mimic this effect by massaging the breasts and gently rolling the nipples between the fingers before expressing and several times throughout the day.

A nasal hormone (oxytocin) spray has been used in a number of hospitals to aid the 'let-down' reflex, and increase the volume of milk produced. The neonatal unit or your family doctor can prescribe this if it seems appropriate. Rest assured that your baby will not go hungry if you do not have enough milk; banked donor milk or formula milk can be given as well.

Relactation

Some mothers only decide that they want to breast-feed when the baby begins to make progress and they are certain he will survive. Others have been given 'drying up' medication in the first day because it was not thought they would want to nurse the baby.

With determination and patience it is possible to build up a milk supply starting weeks or even months after the birth. Very frequent feeds, and nasal oxytocin, may be necessary to stimulate milk production. An ingenious device called Lact-aid has been used by adoptive mothers. This sac and tube fits under the breast and delivers formula milk (or expressed milk) as the baby sucks on the breast, thus providing stimulation to the breasts while satiating the baby's hunger. Giving a tube-feed while the baby is suckling at the breast can mimic this effect too.

The art of sucking

There are a group of reflexes in the full-term infant which help him to learn to suck from the breast or bottle. The first is the 'rooting' reflex; when the corner of his mouth is stroked he turns in that direction, opens his mouth wide, and attempts to latch on to the nipple. The sucking reflex consists of drawing the nipple into his mouth and stripping it with an even pressure at a regular rate. When he is sucking in and swallowing milk he must stop breathing and close off his windpipe (trachea) so that he does not inhale the milk into his lungs.

These reflexes are difficult to elicit in babies of less than 32 weeks gestation. Learning to co-ordinate each component of the process may not happen until after 34–35 weeks. Babies who have had respiratory problems requiring ventilation with an endotracheal tube sometimes have more difficulty learning to feed. They may push the teat out of their mouth with their tongues just as they were trying to do with the tube. At the beginning a preterm baby may clamp onto the nipple or bottle teat but may do little else. Gradually he may make a few sucking movements and then give up.

In the full-term infant a sucking pattern can be demonstrated in which the baby makes a series of sucking movements, then pauses, sucks for a while again, and so on. This is known as a 'burst-pause' pattern. When he is sucking for nourishment, rather than on his fingers, the sucking bursts may go on for more than a minute before a pause. Studies have suggested that individual babies have their own unique patterns of sucking which are fairly consistent over time. In preterm babies these patterns may not be apparent. At the beginning of his sucking experience the preterm baby may suck in an irregular and disorganized way, stopping to rest because he tires more easily, or pausing to breathe and swallow because he cannot co-ordinate these other two actions with his sucking. By 36–38 weeks gestation his sucking skills are becoming similar to those of full-term babies. We still do not know how much these feeding abilities depend on maturation of the reflexes and whether learning and practice can accelerate them.

Starting to suck

To the mother of a full-term baby the first feed may be just part and parcel of caretaking in the early days. In contrast the mother of a preterm baby can often remember to the minute the first time she gave her baby a bottle, or put him to the breast. If he was very small or sick at birth the parents may regard his first 'feed' as a real milestone—a signal that he is now 'stable' enough to tolerate a prolonged period out of the incubator, 'strong' enough to be allowed to try sucking, and 'mature' enough to be able to draw in and swallow the milk.

It may come as a surprise then that there are not usually set criteria which determine when this important event should be allowed. Obviously it is dependent on a baby's medical condition to some extent, and some units may have a minimum weight or gestation criterion. However, the most common 'reason' for giving a baby this opportunity is that he seems 'ready to suck', meaning

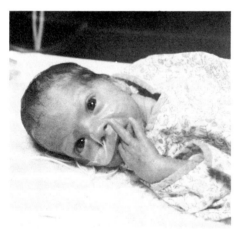

Sometimes sucking on her own fingers may be taken as an indication that she is ready to try breast or bottle feeding.

that he is occasionally observed to suck on his fingers, or tries to suck on his mother's or the nurse's finger.

Many small babies do get tired quickly, so do not expect too much at first; just enjoy cuddling him close to you. The staff will advise you on how long to continue in the early stages. As his stamina increases you will be able to let him suck for as long as he wants, and increasingly frequently.

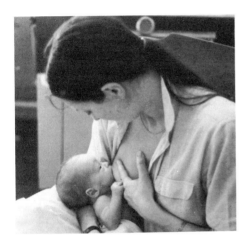

Many mothers come to successfully breast-feed their preterm babies, but it may take many weeks before breast-feeding is established and some mothers, for no lack of trying, find themselves unable to achieve it as the sole source of their baby's nutrition.

A baby may have difficulty in attaching (latching on) to the breast if he tends to put his tongue to the roof of his mouth. Depressing his chin or tongue with a finger passed into his mouth, as you are placing your baby on your breast, may get round this problem.

While in hospital you can be with your baby a lot of the time. If you are discharged home before your baby is ready to leave the neonatal unit demand feeding (feeding the baby when he is ready for a feed) may not be possible at first. You should still visit him often since successful breast-feeding depends to a great extent on getting as much practice as possible. For those feeds when you are not there your baby will probably be tube-fed with your expressed breast-milk.

Sometimes it is quite difficult to provide enough milk by expressing and so your baby will receive donor milk, or some formula feeds, as well as the milk you provide. You should not be discouraged by this since, as time goes by, the amount of milk you provide is likely to increase and will come to be quite sufficient for your baby's needs. However this stage may not be reached until both you and your baby have gone home.

Making progress

When your baby does seem ready for the bottle or breast these will be introduced gradually. He will probably start with one feed a day for a few days to see that he does not choke on the milk, or become overtired. He will then progress to being given several opportunities each day, followed by alternate feeds, and finally by complete breast- or bottle-feeding.

Some babies tolerate this schedule quite well and quickly learn what feeding is all about. Others seem to 'forget' what to do between feeds, particularly when their sucking experience is limited to once a day. With the agreement of medical staff it may be better to give your baby a few minutes of sucking experience before each tube feed so that he gets practice several times a day rather than during one long session.

A few places have given their babies a dummy (pacifier) to suck while they are being tube-fed in order to help establish the co-ordination of sucking skills before having to swallow milk at the same time. Although different strategies are required for feeding from the breast or an artificial teat, it may be that any sucking experience in preterms is valuable in promoting the complex skills involved.

Some preterm babies find it rather difficult to suck from the large, firm, bottle teats (nipples) that are usually available for full-term babies in hospital. A number of manufacturers now produce smaller, softer, teats that may suit your baby better; in America these are widely available in local shops. A variety of 'orthodontic' teats, shaped more like a human nipple, and designed to encourage 'oral exercise', and the correct alignment of later teeth and jaw formation, are also popular there. The build-up of a vacuum in the bottle during feeding can also cause problems for the preterm baby. Some mothers have found it useful to use one of the 'collapsible bag' bottles where this does not occur.

'He just isn't interested!'—Waking the sleepy baby

This is probably the most frequent 'complaint' from mothers whose baby is beginning to suck from the breast or bottle. The baby may never really wake up during the feed, or he may doze off halfway through, or he may make only feeble sucking attempts throughout a lengthy feeding session. This is both disappointing and exasperating for a mother, who may soon begin to feel that her own milk supply is 'inadequate', or that her technique (either breast or bottle) is 'all wrong'.

There is rarely a single obvious cause for this state of affairs. For instance, some preterm infants are rather drowsy and lethargic until they reach a chronological gestation of 37–38 weeks. Your baby may, by temperament, simply be a sleepy, placid kind of baby, or the feedtimes, arranged for the benefit of nursing rotas, may not actually agree with *his* sleep cycle!

There are many ways of trying to wake a sleeping baby, and finding out which are successful with *your* baby takes time and

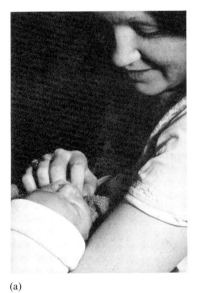
(a)

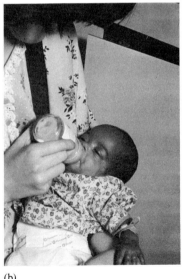
(b)

(a) Stroking his chin and around his mouth may help to wake the baby for his feed.

(b) When cuddled close there is no reason why giving a bottle-feed can't be just as rewarding for both mother and baby as breast-feeding.

practice. It may help to establish a consistent kind of signal to the baby that it is feeding time; loosening his blankets, unwrapping him and changing his nappy (diaper) may rouse him. If not, stroking his hands, tickling his feet, talking to him, and putting him upright over your shoulder, may work. Eliciting the rooting reflex, or rubbing his back or forehead, can serve as preparatory signs that you have come to feed him.

The days and weeks of waiting for your baby to become fully competent at feeding can seem never-ending. A baby of 32 weeks or less may be expected to take several weeks between his first taste of milk, and finishing every feed. It is easy to become discouraged by the many ups and downs during this time. One day your baby may drink most of every bottle, or suckle happily for 30 minutes on the breast, and then the next he may steadfastly refuse to suck at all. Some days his weight will be static, and then he will suddenly make-up for lost time with a large gain.

Hospital support for breast-feeding

It is sad that breast-feeding is often more difficult in the hospital environment. Mothers who want to breast-feed their baby—full-term or preterm—can experience problems in establishing lactation, and may not enjoy what should be a satisfying and rewarding activity. The mother whose baby is in a neonatal unit has particular problems to overcome, not least because she will be concerned that he takes enough milk to thrive, and because it is difficult to feel 'at home' in such a bustling, noisy, and public environment. There are a number of things which can help promote successful breast-feeding—and for that matter bottle-feeding—in preterm babies:

(1) accurate and consistent advice about feeding from the nursing staff, particularly from staff who have breast-fed a baby themselves,

(2) provision of privacy (a separate room, or screens at least) and comfort (rocking chairs, supportive back pillows, rubber rings, or inflatable cushions to ease the discomfort of stitches),

(3) availability of efficient and reliable breast-pumping systems so that a mother can express milk until her baby is ready to suckle, and even then to provide milk for the feeds when she cannot visit,

(4) flexible routines which can meet the individual needs of both the baby and his mother. For instance, some 31 week gestation babies are ready to suck under supervision; in others tube and breast-feeding simultaneously may encourage the reluctant feeder. Sometimes a mother may prefer to go home breast-feeding but with bottle supplements, and this should be respected too.

To finally hold the baby in their arms and feed him—be it by bottle or breast—is often the most memorable event for parents during their baby's stay in hospital. Their many comments indicate that meeting this need themselves marks the transition to what they see as the beginning of real parenthood

'Scary at times . . . as she had some apnoeic attacks'

'Difficult at first—I felt detached—it was like feeding the nurses' baby. Now it is perfect.'

'It was interesting to see how he took it as he was so small.'

'Joy being able to participate after being separated for so long.'

'It was fantastic to breast-feed my baby after having to tube-feed her for so long.'

'Great . . . lovely . . . Now she's really mine.'

8

Even small babies are clever: how a preterm baby behaves

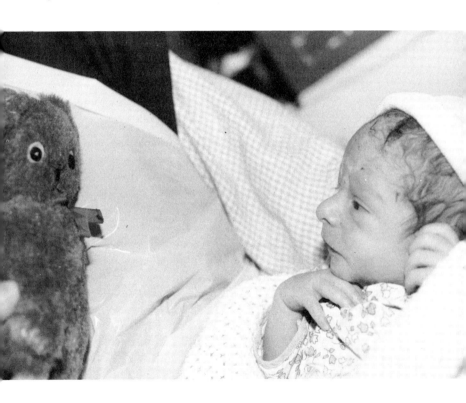

It is hard to believe that a newly-born preterm baby, attached to equipment to assist his breathing and to an array of monitoring devices, could possibly be involved in anything beyond his immediate physiological needs. Indeed, only in recent years has it become acknowledged that newborn full-term infants rather than being 'helpless little bundles' can be active and responsive participants, interested in both the physical and social world into which they have just been born. Old wives' tales persist, books about child care and parenting are not always up to date, and even some medical personnel still believe that newborn babies cannot see, and that during the early weeks they can only respond to light and dark. For parents of preterm babies these widely held views make the task of getting to know their baby seem a daunting, if not impossible one.

Research and observation have shown that normal full-term babies can see and hear, detect differences in taste and smell, and be responsive to touch and movement. These abilities enable them to respond to their parents at, or soon after, birth. At full-term the transition from uterus to parents' arms, although a major upheaval, is uncomplicated compared with the situation in which a preterm infant finds himself.

Inside the mother

Within the uterus the growing fetus is exposed to many stimuli: he can react to the taste of different substances introduced into the amniotic fluid, detect changes in light and darkness, hear loud noises from outside, and is exposed to a great many more from within; these include the sounds of blood circulating, his mother's heartbeat, her breathing, and movements in her digestive tract. The fetus himself makes periodic breathing movements, sucks on his fingers, and punches and kicks. He can be seen on ultrasound scans to make both small and large postural adjustments. However in the fluid medium in which he grows the effect of gravity is diminished; floating in amniotic fluid makes moving easier and, at the same time, has the effect of damping down the violence of all movements. In the uterus the growing baby is also subjected to his mother's own biological rhythms; her pattern of sleep, wakefulness, activity, and rest, has a regulatory influence on the baby and his activity. This diurnal rhythm of rest and activity, changing over the 24 hours, seems to provide a model for the baby's own behaviour as he is rocked vigorously, or gently, depending on what his mother is doing at the time.

The different experiences of full-term and preterm babies

Life outside is very different. The maturity of full-term babies enables them to cope better with the transition and to begin responding to their new environment. Preterm babies, initially at least, have higher energy needs, and so have little left over for such activities. In contrast to the cushioned environment of the mother's body, a preterm infant is usually nursed on a relatively firm, stationary, surface. Sounds are no longer muffled and familiar; some are constant, like the hum of the incubator motor, or the regular 'bleeps' of the monitoring equipment; others, like the loud, sudden, monitor alarms, occur erratically and unexpectedly. The continuous bright lights of a neonatal unit cause many newborns to keep their eyes closed.

Some psychologists and paediatricians consider this environment to be one of sensory 'bombardment', while others think that the lack of structured and meaningful stimuli constitutes a form of 'sensory deprivation'. In reality it is probably a mixture of both. The high level of technology required to support the lives of some babies born before their expected time does indeed result in what can only be described as a highly artificial environment in which to live and grow. A baby's needs for nutrition, oxygen, and assistance in temperature regulation, once supplied by the mother's body, must now be met by a complicated array of equipment and procedures administered by highly trained personnel. It is these which contribute to the contrast between neonatal units and home, or postnatal wards.

Though a preterm baby's experience is clearly different from that of babies born at term many are responsive to aspects of their new situation. Like full-term babies they are not just passive recipients of the attentions of medical staff and parents. As with other babies not only are there large individual variations in behaviour and responsiveness, but a given baby varies from day to day in how he or she may react, even in what seem to be identical circumstances. Babies born as much as three months early, provide us with an 'experiment of nature'; they give us a valuable window on the last few months of pregnancy that we would not otherwise have. In watching their behaviour and reactions, even in a neonatal unit, it is possible to see that they are not as helpless and unresponsive as might be thought.

Alertness

Even very small babies can pay attention to some of the things happening around them. However, early on, due to fatigue, their periods of alertness may be very brief. With increasing gestational age they are alert more often and for longer periods. Wakefulness may then occur quite spontaneously, rather than just as a result of being handled by nursing staff, or cuddled by their parents.

A preterm baby can give the impression that he would actually prefer to be left alone; he may seem stressed by contact and handling. In time he develops the ability to tolerate 'interference', and to respond positively, revealing a need for people and the kind of contact that they can give. Human contact and an interesting environment become essential requirements for his development.

What is noticeable in some preterm babies, especially the younger ones, is that at times, although their eyes may be wide open and they appear alert they seem out of reach and preoccupied with something of interest in the 'middle distance'. This apparent inattentiveness gradually disappears so that by term they behave more like babies born at full gestation.

Seeing and hearing

Researchers testing the visual behaviour of a large group of preterm babies found at least one baby of less than 30 weeks' gestation who could focus. All but one of the babies examined at 33 weeks not only did this, but also began to follow the movement of a slowly moving object by adjusting the position of their eyes or head. By 34 weeks post-menstrual age most preterm babies showed a fully mature pattern of visual behaviour comparable to that observed in full-term babies; they were clearly able to observe the movement of an object by turning their head and eyes in the correct direction and following it. They could do this whether the object was moved horizontally or vertically.

This perhaps surprising finding, which has since been confirmed,

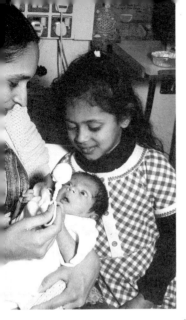
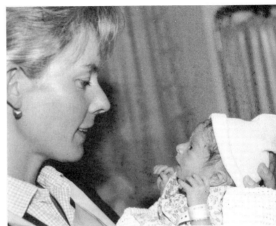

By 32 weeks' gestation, many preterm babies show a keen interest in faces and objects nearby.

should encourage neonatal staff and parents to be attentive to this aspect of preterm infant behaviour. It must be noted however that to obtain these results the babies were propped up at an angle of 30°, the background lighting was turned down, and the object used for testing (a bright red woolly ball) was held only seven inches away. With increasing age and further maturation of the visual system, the optimal viewing distance increases slightly so that normal full-term babies focus on objects *between eight and fifteen inches* away. This process of maturation continues so that at a few weeks of age a baby born at term can usually focus and follow the movement of things that are close, and of those at the far side of the room. Full-term and preterm babies are not just attracted to brightly coloured toys but are very responsive to the human face at the close distances mentioned above. They will often scan a face, showing particular interest in the eyes and hairline as well as in the mouth, especially if the person is speaking to them and making exaggerated lip movements as people often do when talking to young babies. Some infants in fact show a preference for faces rather than inanimate objects or toys. Similarly, a few babies may react more to a human voice than to rattles, musical boxes, or other inanimate sounds.

Sometimes when there is a loud noise outside, a pregnant mother

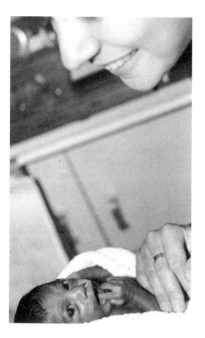

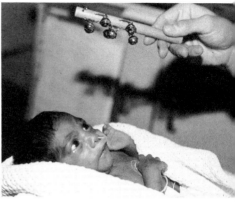

A baby by 33 weeks' gestation shows interest in human voices, rattles, and musical toys.

may feel her baby jump or startle in response to it. But since a mother may also react herself it can be difficult to decide whether the baby is reacting to her surprise or to the sound itself. Reseachers have found heart-rate changes in some babies reacting to noises from outside the uterus, but these seem difficult to obtain consistently, and individual babies react differently. Although there may be little outward sign of auditory responsiveness in the preterm baby after birth, brainwave changes in those parts of the brain which process sounds have been noted as early as 25 weeks gestation after exposure to sounds. By 28 weeks a few preterm babies have been found to respond to the noise of a rattle by searching around with their eyes, and even by turning in the direction of the sound, but this is unusual. More commonly, by about 33 weeks, most seem to listen, and then turn their heads towards the source of the noise to left or right as appropriate; this is regardless of whether the sound is a rattle or human voice. The voice needs to be loud and varying in pitch to obtain an optimal response.

The speed and reliability of these responses to sights and sounds gradually improves with time, but that they should occur at all in preterm babies is in many ways remarkable. This responsiveness is reduced when a baby is ill or has a set-back. Babies with medical problems may be slower or more variable in their responses, and some may not seem to react at all, though their heart and respiration rates may show changes. Once an ill preterm baby is recovering he becomes more able to deal with the outside world and to make use of these abilities.

Sucking and rooting behaviour

The natural response of a full-term baby when the area of his cheek near the corner of his mouth is touched is to turn his head in the direction of the stimulus, while opening his mouth and attempting to latch on to what would be his mother's breast. This reaction, which is an important part of feeding behaviour, is called the 'rooting reflex'. Before 32 weeks gestation very few babies show this behaviour, and those that do are usually slow to respond. Between 33–36 weeks of gestational age they improve, becoming quicker and more efficient, so that by 40 weeks their rooting reflex seems little different from that of full-term babies.

The 'sucking reflex', like rooting, is really primed to work better nearer to full gestation. It is however a more complicated behaviour and thus more liable to suffer disruption when a baby is born too soon. The co-ordination of sucking, swallowing, and breathing, which is necessary for feeding, is even more complex and more of an effort than the finger-sucking a baby may have been practising before birth. Normal full-term babies vary considerably in their ability to co-ordinate these reflexes and may take a few days to learn to do so.

As was discussed in Chapter 7, all babies, including those who have been born prematurely, suck in a 'burst-pause' kind of pattern. This means that they make a series of sucking movements, have a pause, suck more, pause again and so on. There is great variation between individual babies in how fast they suck, in how long the sucking bursts are, and in the length of the pauses in between. Early on, a preterm baby may just clamp onto the nipple or bottle teat and show little inclination to suck at all. By 40 weeks a preterm baby may still not be as efficient at feeding as a full-term baby, but with more time and experience this difference disappears.

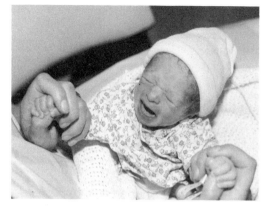

A crying baby is comforted by being held and talked to; he quiets and, in th[?] instance, becomes alert to his caregive[?]

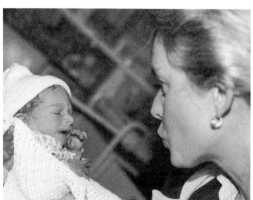

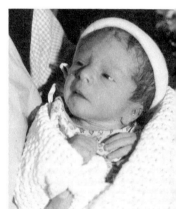

Crying

Many young preterm babies cry infrequently, if at all. This contributes to the great difference between the noise in a neonatal unit and that heard on a typical hospital postnatal ward. Instead of the loud cries of many babies, there is the sound of monitors, and the conversation of staff and parents. In contrast to the loud vigorous cries or screams of full-term babies, preterm babies seem to fuss, whimper, or 'whine'; muffled by the incubator walls, these weak cries are scarcely audible.

Once a preterm baby has grown bigger and stronger he is more likely to cry spontaneously, as well as in response to handling. By about 36 weeks these babies seem to have more energy, crying frequently and on less provocation than before. They may need more assistance in the form of talking and holding to help them settle down again after they have been upset. This more frequent crying is often preceded by an increase in fussiness between about 33 and 35 weeks gestation. To parents that have had a small preterm baby it may seem that just as he appears to be well and growing he starts becoming fussy and difficult to manage. The contrast with the previous quietness and lack of responsiveness contributes to this feeling, as does the fact that parents with a baby in special care have had less chance to get to know their baby. Direct comparison of full-term and preterm babies at 40 weeks post-menstrual age does reveal that full-term babies may actually cry more, and that they do so in response to milder stimuli; they can have more difficulty in quietening themselves than babies born prematurely. Once home the situation may change with an older preterm baby crying more loudly and more often (see Chapter 12).

It seems that the use of crying as a signal, and the development of different kinds of cry, are signs of increasing maturity and to be expected in a growing preterm baby, even if not actually welcomed. When a preterm baby cries he may be hungry, or uncomfortable, and need feeding or changing. Boredom can result in crying, and some enjoy being carried around, played with, and entertained. Others simply seem to need a loving cuddle.

Sleeping and waking

During pregnancy most mothers are aware that the baby they are carrying has definite periods of activity and rest. These may not always coincide with the mother's own pattern of activity but, nevertheless, will to some degree be conditioned by it. Once birth has taken place this organizing influence is lost, and clearly a preterm baby will have had less experience in this respect than one born at term. Observations of preterm babies indicate that they tend to have a less organized pattern of sleeping and waking than term infants. This may be partly due to the lack of maternal rhythms and to the fact that in the neonatal unit environment, especially that of intensive care, a baby may be woken at frequent intervals so that necessary medical and nursing procedures can be carried out. In such circumstances the difference between day and night is minimized and babies are fed according to schedule, so it may be quite difficult for a baby to develop his own individual pattern.

Most newborn babies sleep a good deal, and preterm babies perhaps more so. The younger they are in terms of gestational age the more likely this is to be the case. Babies of less than 32 weeks' gestation very often remain asleep even during caretaking routines, and when having a cuddle. But a week or so later they may wake as their position is altered, their nappy changed, or as they are picked up and talked to. Even so it must be remembered that there are large individual differences; some babies tire more easily than others. There are also large day to day variations in the way a particular baby behaves. Preterm babies especially, can find even simple medical procedures like being weighed or having a blood sample taken very exhausting, and quickly fall asleep afterwards. By 38 weeks however, the amount of time spent sleeping is similar to that observed in full-term babies, though of course, like them, this may be considerably less than their parents had anticipated.

While asleep it is important for a baby to be able to 'tune' out and ignore irrelevant noises and lights; this process is called 'habituation'. The first responses of a sleeping baby to an unexpected light or sound may be to blink and startle, change his breathing, and move his arms and legs, but with each successive presentation of the light or sound the baby reacts less, and finally not at all. This protective behaviour which allows a baby to stay asleep despite the noises and activity going on around him, is something that most full-term babies are capable of to a varying degree.

At around 28 weeks gestation preterm babies can begin to habituate to sounds, but when a light is quickly shone on and off their faces they tend to close their eyes for half a minute or more. By 32 weeks they react more appropriately closing their eyes for a shorter time. Right up to 40 weeks post-menstrual age preterm babies seem to be better at ignoring irrelevant sounds than irrelevant lights, despite being looked after in the brightly lit world of the neonatal unit. The ability to habituate to redundant or irrelevant sights and sounds while asleep improves as a baby gets older. Responses become rapid and brief with little or no body or limb movement. By 40 weeks, babies born prematurely behave little differently from those that are newly-born at term, in spite of their very different experiences.

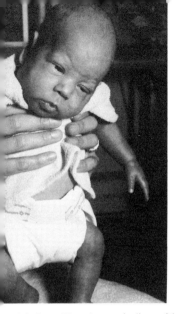
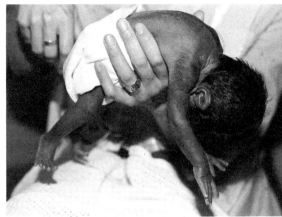

A baby at 35 weeks may be limp with poor tone and has poor head control with little ability to support his body weight.

Activity and movement

Young preterm infants tend to be relatively inactive. When they are active the immature movements look restricted and jerky. Gradually, with maturation, overall activity increases and the movements become bigger and smoother.

Preterm babies of less than 32 weeks gestation may seem limp and floppy a lot of the time. There may be little resistance when their limbs are moved, and spontaneous movements are erratic and often tremulous (jittery). It is the presence of muscle 'tone' which increases with age that gives rise to this resistance. Preterm babies tend to have sudden fluctuations in tone while being handled. This means that at one moment they may seem quite tense, even stiff, while at the next they may be quite limp and flaccid. By about 38 weeks gestation they are more likely to respond by increasing their muscle tone when handled.

In the uterus, the cramped position of late pregnancy provides a different experience for a baby born at term compared with the lack of constraint provided by the preterm baby's incubator or cot. On reaching 40 weeks gestational age a preterm baby is more likely to have 'extended' or straightened legs when being examined, whereas a full-term baby's legs are 'flexed' or bent. This difference is quite normal and not thought to be of medical significance. At

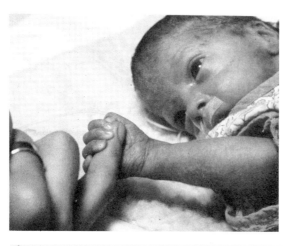

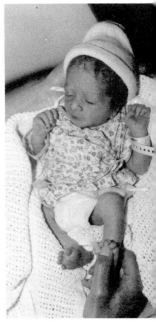

Reflex responses to placing an object in the hand or under the toe cause grasping; allowing the head to fall gently backwards initiates the Moro response with extension of arms and fingers followed by movement of the arms across the body.

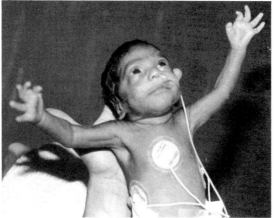

40 weeks a preterm baby's head and trunk control may be better than that of a full-term baby for he has had a chance to practise supporting his head and coping with the full effects of gravity for sometime.

The lack of space in the uterus which encourages the flexed (curled up) posture of full-term babies also results in a closer proximity between hands and mouth enabling them to suck on their fingers. Preterm babies may necessarily be nursed in positions which are not conducive to this kind of behaviour, and do seem less able in this respect. Though they improve over time and make brief swipes with a hand near their mouth, even at 40 weeks gestational age they rarely manage to place a hand in the mouth and keep it there. This activity is important as it is one way for a baby to quiet himself, and stay alert, and look around without fussing, or to go to sleep peacefully.

Perhaps because they are generally more fatigued and need to conserve their limited energy resources, young very preterm babies have less jittery or tremulous movements, and fewer startles than their older counterparts. These reactions seem to increase in number up to 35 weeks' gestation and then to decline so that at around 40 weeks most preterm babies jump or startle as much, and show a similar amount of tremor, to that seen in normal babies born at the usual time.

Some reflex patterns seem to develop in a preterm baby much as they would have done had the baby continued to grow in the mother's uterus. Others appears to be affected by the very different experiences these babies have. Walking and crawling reflexes, despite the chance of practising on the incubator mattress, or on the laps of parents and nursing staff, are less well developed at 40 weeks post-menstrual age than in full-term newborns. However the 'palmar' (hand) grasp, which is weaker and more variable in young preterm babies, shows increasing promptness and efficiency with increasing age, so that at 40 weeks many preterm babies grasp and hold onto a finger with as much strength as any full-term infant.

Demonstrating babies' skills

Formal studies by psychologists on the behavioural development of preterm babies can provide useful information for parents and medical staff. Giving parents feedback about their baby's developing abilities helps them to know what to expect of their baby, and confirms their own experience gained from watching and handling him. Demonstrating his responses to voices and faces, and his range of movements such as head turning, standing with support, and toe and finger grasping, gives them more confidence in their involvement with him.

The fragile appearance of preterm babies makes many parents very tentative in their efforts to touch and hold their baby. Showing them how well their baby tolerates being placed prone (on his tummy) or being 'pulled to sit' can give them the reassurance they need, and enhance their enjoyment of the baby.

Nurses, too, need to be aware of the developing skills of preterm infants. This can make care-giving more rewarding, as well as enabling them to guide parents through some of the more demanding and difficult periods their baby may experience: for example at times when he is unresponsive, and later on when he may become overfussy.

Maximizing early development: what can be done to help?

The behaviour and development of preterm babies are influenced by many complex and often interrelated factors. Individual differences in temperament which can be evident even at this early stage, different nursing procedures, and the severity of particular medical complications, all affect the way a baby behaves. In spite of these difficulties, and the contrast between being cared for in a neonatal unit and continuing to grow in utero, many preterm babies do show that they have a great ability to overcome the disadvantage. They show more resilience than many people, including some professionals, would credit them with.

Direct comparison of the two environments can create a rather negative picture, but it is necessary to be realistic about what a preterm baby is missing out on and to try and understand the stresses that he typically experiences. Parents need to understand why their babies look and behave as they do.

Over the last decade or so, as survival rates for small preterm babies have improved, researchers have described their early development and tried to identify their particular needs at this time. Being cared for in hospital in an open crib, or in an incubator, a child is, to a great extent, isolated from human contact and separated from his parents. Apart from attempts to increase human contact one approach in trying to minimize the differences has been to mimic some of the features of the uterine environment. To this end light levels have been reduced, babies have been nursed on water beds with a built-in oscillation that is based on the timing of a mother's breathing movements and sound recordings of a mother's heart beat, and of actual noises recorded in the uterus ('womb music'), have been played to them. Another approach has been to provide different forms of stimulation and 'enrichment'. These have included the provision of lambs' wool to lie on as an alternative to the usual cotton bedding, the use of stroking or

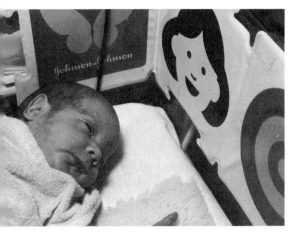

Images of high contrast placed close to a baby provide a stimulating environment which interests her.

massage techniques applied daily or several times a day, dummies or 'pacifiers' to suck on, and visual excitement in the form of pictures and musical toys made of contrasting brightly coloured materials.

The objectives are twofold—to give a preterm baby perceptual stimulation when awake, and to help reduce fussing and crying and the associated uncoordinated, wasteful, erratic movements. As a result babies in 'intervention programmes' which use these techniques, have often been found to gain weight better, and to be more responsive and alert than those receiving normal care. Some paediatricians are now taking up these research findings and are changing their procedures and practices. However, it should be noted that some preterm babies can be 'overloaded' and care must be taken in choosing the form of stimulation, and the time at which it is used, for the individual baby.

A key feature of the special care experience, especially that of intensive care, is the arbitrary nature of the stimulation which a baby may receive. Little of it is 'contingent', that is dependent on what a baby is doing. A tube-feed may be given when a baby is asleep rather than when he's awake, and a radio or cassette recorder playing music most of the time may alleviate staff boredom or make parents feel more relaxed, but it does little for the babies, who have no control over it. However by arranging things so that a water bed rocks only when a baby is moving or crying, or that a musical mobile plays only when a baby is awake, stimulation can be made more meaningful for the baby. The most appropriate form of stimulation usually comes when parents visit. They are likely to have more time and motivation than the busy nursing staff caring for many different babies, and be able to wait for their baby to wake naturally. As they gain confidence during their visits they come to talk to, touch, and stroke, cuddle and rock their baby, so the presence of parents in the hospital where their preterm baby is being cared for is not just desirable but necessary, both from their own point of view, and for the benefit of the baby. As awareness of the baby's responsiveness increases, when her baby waves an arm or stretches, his mother may smile; when his baby's eyes open and focus, the father may move up close and talk with his baby; when the baby cries either parent may try out ways of comforting him by touching and stroking, swaddling, cuddling, or rocking him, as his condition permits. When parents behave in these ways their baby's senses are stimulated in an appropriate, rather than in an arbitrary, or chance, fashion.

Practical aspects of promoting early interaction

'Don't rush him'; 'Take your time'—these maxims should be in parents' minds during the early months. Each baby has a style of reacting to events going on round him and responds at a pace which suits him. Give him time to 'warm up', and to look at and listen to what you are doing and saying. Then let him have his turn at responding—to look, smile, or move his arms and legs—and give him time. By four months post-term many mothers and their infants are so in harmony that each partner can be seen making her own moves as well as anticipating the other's next.

Studies of mothers and their preterm infants have indicated that because these immature babies make fewer demands and responses most new moves and initiatives come from the mothers; they take over both active roles in the 'conversation'—initiating and responding. This can rob a baby of his earliest opportunities to develop a level of autonomy—to gradually become aware of his own relevance in giving happiness and causing other reactions in his caregivers.

It is more effective with a sick or preterm baby to work through a repertoire of items which rouse him gently rather than to begin by talking loudly, waving a rattle, or doing both at once. Talk softly from one side and bring your face close to his and wait. He may squirm, open an eye, or startle, and only then become interested. It is not unusual for a preterm baby to end the 'conversation' by becoming jittery, slightly blue, or breathless. These are signals that he needs a short rest to regain his equilibrium. In time he becomes more able to cope with the ever increasing bombardment of stimuli from the world outside, as a consequence of his steadily maturing nervous system.

In summary, preterm babies, though not always initially as responsive as babies born at full-term, come to show that they can hear, see, and respond to their new physical and social environment. The exact way in which they react will depend on their particular circumstances, and will alter as they grow and develop. In caring for babies who have been born prematurely a situation is aimed at in which there is a balance between medical necessities and psychological needs. For each baby the situation is different, and in every intensive care centre and neonatal unit, as practices and technology advance, so will this balance change.

9
Parents' feelings

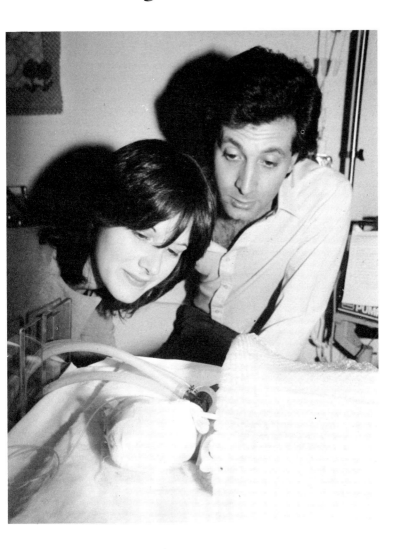

Preterm birth is a crisis event and crises precipitate a range of responses in different individuals. Most often parents are shocked, finding it hard to believe that this could have happened to them. As they look back on this period of their lives, it is typically remembered as a nightmare of lights and equipment where their baby was barely visible.

Not only does a preterm birth prevent parents from making the usual plans and preparations that are normally part of the last weeks of pregnancy, but it also deprives them of an important time together for making psychological adjustments before the baby arrives. Parents in this situation have to cope with a small, possibly ill baby, who looks very unlike the large, well-rounded, healthy infant they were led to expect would be theirs.

Early days

Initially, though shocked, parents experience a mixture of many emotions. Exactly which, and in what proportion, will depend on their particular personalities, backgrounds, and life experiences. They are likely to be very disappointed that the pregnancy did not continue for the full nine months, even if this has happened to them before. At the same time they may feel guilty that in some way they have been responsible for the fact that their baby was born too soon. Mothers of preterm babies feel that they, or their bodies, have been at fault. Fathers may blame their partner, but generally they are simply upset and angry that this should have happened. Sometimes they seek to blame some event or medical procedure from the recent, or even quite distant, past.

Both parents may be horrified at the appearance of their baby, especially if very immature. Some have said that he looked like 'a skinned rabbit', or seemed 'more like an ugly little doll', than a proper baby. 'The baby seemed unfinished' is a commonly expressed sentiment. Such feelings need to be acknowledged as quite reasonable in the circumstances, for parents can feel guilty about these too. They may also be aware of feelings of rejection at this stage because this baby was not the one they had wanted.

Just as they are presented with a baby who is very unlike the one they had expected, parents are confronted with the possibility of his needing intensive or special medical care. They fear that he could die at any moment. Parents are considerably frightened by the fragile appearance of their preterm baby and the apparently tenuous hold on life which he has, as emphasised by all the equipment being used to keep him alive. Many, already distressed at being separated from their baby, and at having missed out on the experience of a normal birth, become detached at this time. 'I held back', 'I didn't want to get too close to her', and 'I didn't want to get too involved', are typical of the remarks parents make about this period.

The need to nurture and care for their baby has been thwarted, and there are few incentives to visit and make contact with a baby who may not live to become a full member of the family. This 'anticipatory grief' reaction is one that is commonly experienced by mothers and fathers of babies who are sick or premature. Sadly, at this stage parents are very often unable to discuss their worst fears with each other. At such an obviously worrying time they may try to buoy each other up with assumed cheerfulness and well-being. Encouraging comments to each other like 'Of course he'll be all right', and 'They can do wonders nowadays', are made without a great deal of confidence or certainty. Some couples are drawn together by the experience and their relationship strengthened, but until their baby's medical condition has stabilized they may still find it hard to discuss their feelings about the situation.

During the early days, each time a parent telephones the neonatal intensive care unit to ask how their baby is getting on, or as they walk down the hospital corridors on their way to visit the baby, they feel apprehensive and concerned that something dreadful may have happened in their absence. In trying to prepare for the worst, and in attempting to avoid the hurt and disappointment that might come, they distance themselves from the situation. For some parents it is as if they cannot afford the emotional investment of becoming deeply attached to a small, sick, baby. As a result it is hard for them to follow the advice of the unit staff to visit frequently, and to touch or stroke their baby. Those parents who do wish to have contact with their baby, despite the off-putting technology, and his worrying appearance, feel that there is little they can do in comparison with the nursing care given by experienced professionals. When parents do manage to reach in to the incubator and hold or stroke their baby's hand they may find themselves inhibited by the presence of other parents or staff, and the general lack of privacy that prevails in most intensive care units. It is difficult to time visits to fit in with a baby's activity periods, and many parents say that they feel foolish sitting in front of an incubator in which an infant is sleeping quietly. When a baby is born very early, or is ill, parents may spend prolonged periods staring at the small rib cage heaving up and down and listening to the bleeps and alarm bells from monitoring equipment. They snatch quick glances at the visual display units which show respiration and heart rates, and soon learn the significance of any changes. For nearly all parents this is an extremely stressful experience which many will have to go through time and again until their baby's particular medical problems have been overcome. Bradycardias and apnoeic episodes can cause them much concern. The unfamiliar, highly technical environment of intensive care, coupled with the enforced separation which comes with it, can conspire to make parents feel inadequate, irrelevant and useless. Not only were they unable to have a normal baby like most other people, but now they are not even able to look after him themselves.

Some parents find it hard to express just how anxious they feel at this point, and may stop visiting altogether. A few suppress their feelings to the extent of not being conscious of their anxieties at all; this may come over to staff as an unwarrantedly carefree attitude, or as overt cheerfulness when the baby's condition would be expected to cause concern. Such parental reactions may indicate underlying psychological problems, but more frequently represent an extreme way of coping with fear and uncertainty. Providing them with opportunities to talk privately with a paediatrician about the baby can often bring relief and a more realistic appreciation of the baby's condition and likely pattern of recovery. Parents who continue to react to the crisis of a preterm birth by 'denying' their feelings may benefit from short-term psychiatric support.

A great deal of tactful and supportive care by nurses and doctors is required to help parents through this period. Many parents with a preterm baby are themselves in need of this kind of 'special care', but not all staff find themselves able to adopt a nurturant attitude towards them. This may be a consequence not only of individual differences in personality and social skills, but also in the kind of training received. There is usually little course-time set aside for dealing with these problems.

In the environment of the neonatal unit the conditions for getting to know one's own baby are far from ideal. Parents find it hard to watch while painful medical procedures are carried out, and many indeed withdraw from the situation completely, often feeling helpless and guilty in doing so. Those that are present, unless they are unusually detached, feel upset at not being able to prevent these things happening to their baby, and in not being able to comfort the baby sufficiently and make the hurt better. The inability to carry out the normal caring role makes many parents feel frustrated. These feelings may be exacerbated by the apparent slowness of their baby to recover and grow.

When asked about these early days many parents have said that the worst thing about having their baby looked after in a neonatal unit was the lack of contact. 'I was upset because I couldn't feed or even hold him', 'It was painful not having my baby beside me' and 'There was an ache because I was apart from my baby and I was not able to find the bond between her and me', are some of the words parents have used to try and express their feelings about the separation from their baby.

Going home without the baby

Going home without their baby can be traumatic for parents, even though they know he or she is in safe hands. Leaving her baby in hospital makes a mother's feelings of distress and anxiety yet more acute. Many are weepy and unable to stop bursting into tears and say that they feel 'upset', 'depressed', 'empty', and as if 'part of me was missing'.

On the one hand being near the unit may be an encouragement for a mother to stay in hospital. On the other hand if she is put where she can see other babies, or hear their cries, she may prefer to go home. Either way parents may have regrets, and as one mother said 'I wanted to go home because I couldn't face the other mothers with their normal babies, but when I got home I felt depressed and unhappy and wished that I had stayed in hospital'. There is no really good compromise for parents in this situation. Many have practical preparations that they need to make before they are ready for the baby to come home. It is important that mothers do not become 'institutionalized' and that they take up the familiar responsibilities of running their lives again. After the shattering blow to self-esteem that preterm birth can bring, parents need to take steps in rebuilding their self-confidence. Going home and coping with day to day routines is part of this process.

Staff and parents

At the beginning, and at times when things are critical, parents have a clearly dependent relationship with the staff in the hospital. Later, when the situation is more stable and they would like to be involved in their own baby's care, some staff resist giving up part of the caretaking role. A mother particularly may feel that some-how the hospital is denying her contact with her baby, whether or not this is in fact the case. The natural anxiety of most new parents is heightened in these circumstances in which they have no clearly defined role, and in which the majority of their infant's care is necessarily undertaken by highly trained personnel. Uncertainty about what to do when they visit, but feeling they have to come because it is expected of them, even though there is little to occupy the time, places an added strain on parents who are already stressed.

Staff attitudes and expectations can have a very positive effect on parents in helping them to care for, and get to know, their baby. But differences of social class, temperament, and culture, on either side, can lead to misunderstandings which are detrimental to the developing relationship between parents and child. Often parents are aware of how they may have been categorized by staff, some-times on the basis of very little information; some as 'young and irresponsible', others as 'thoughtless and uncaring', or even as 'over-anxious and over-educated'. Such labelling is unlikely to con-tribute to the well-being of any of those concerned, and may gen-erate considerable bad feeling. By getting to know each other as individuals the chances of this happening can be reduced. This may also facilitate the gradual transfer of care from the specially trained nurses to the parents who will actually be bringing the child up.

All the stresses and strains that have been described are likely to have a physical effect on parents. Many mention difficulties in sleeping and eating, and poor concentration, especially fathers while at work. Mothers, particularly those who are hoping to breast-feed, find it hard to cope with the conflicting requests made of them to rest a good deal, and yet to visit frequently.

To start with, mothers and fathers are worried about handling their small babies, fearing that the various tubes, electrical leads, and intravenous drips may become detached or dislodged. Help to overcome such natural fears can be given by experienced members of staff in the form of gentle encouragement, and by telling parents about the equipment in use with their baby. This is particularly important in view of mothers' and fathers' reports that they did not begin to feel the baby belonged to them until they held him in their arms.

Growing and getting better

Once the baby has been moved to a cot and is being monitored less intensively, parents' attitudes and expectations change. Greater involvement in their baby's care means that they can now begin to imagine taking their baby home—something that has been very hard to do up to now. Though they may have been involved in tube-feeding, most mothers prefer to feed their baby in a more conventional manner, and see the transition to breast or bottle, along with the transfer to a cot, as a clear mark of the baby's progress and recovery.

However things do not always go as smoothly as parents had hoped; feeding a small sleepy baby can be time-consuming and frustrating, and weight gain may be slow or erratic. The necessarily more frequent visits to the hospital brought about by the more active participation of parents in caring for their baby, can result in quite a demanding schedule.

For most parents this is a period of readjustment. The detachment that was a defence mechanism earlier is now exchanged for anxiety about the future. Instead of fears of being too involved, some parents now become over-protective to the extent of criticizing staff care, and being jealous of their own partner's contact with the baby.

By this stage a mother has, to some extent, come to terms with 'her failure' to carry her baby for the full gestation. Both she and the baby's father now need to concern themselves with getting to know their baby as an individual. Parents need time and help to see their baby as a growing and changing infant rather than as the small fragile person they first saw. This is a difficult thing to do in what they perceive as an artificial setting. The loss of confidence and self-esteem felt by most parents who have had a premature baby is hard to overcome. Doubting their own abilities, even if they have had a baby before, can make parents self-conscious and shy about taking a more active part in their baby's care. Some worry about their own ability to cope, both now and later, while others feel that they are in the way and something of a nuisance. These feelings can make parents nervous and tentative in handling their baby. At this point particularly many need reassurance that they are doing the right thing, as well as information about the ways in which preterm and full-term babies are different.

Some parents take longer than others to adjust to the transfer of their baby from an incubator to a cot. Delighted initially, they may worry as to whether he can manage without all the apparatus they had got used to seeing. The advantages, for them however, clearly out-weigh these concerns: 'I can give him a cuddle whenever I like now'; 'I don't feel shut off from her any more', and 'It's more what I'm used to, with a nightie, bedclothes and all'.

Most parents feel more at ease once their baby is in a cot, but they can undergo rapid swings of mood, depending on how each visit goes, and how things are at home. A baby who never seems to be awake and alert when parents come, or who is very slow to feed or gain weight, can give rise to feelings of inadequacy and hopelessness. Problems at home, even minor ones, can add to this. Doubting themselves they are likely to feel that they are failures and that the nurses' care must be better. At the same time their feelings can be very mixed and they may at times resent the nursing staff who have contact with their baby. These doubts and worries are exaggerated by the prospect of having to cope on their own with the baby at home.

Going home

Taking their baby home from hospital is a momentous event for all parents, but especially so for those who have had a preterm baby. Some parents feel excited and optimistic about the next few weeks, but others still feel detached and find it hard to believe that they are really going to have their baby to themselves. The bigger the gap between when the baby was born and when he or she is taken home, the more likely the parents are to express feelings of unreality, or to find the responsibility for total care quite over-whelming.

At this stage many parents say that they want to try and make up for all that has happened, even to the extent of giving more as a way of compensating for the bad start their baby had. Delighted to have the baby home at last parents generally find the first few days more tiring than they had expected. Mothers, who usually have a greater responsibility in looking after the baby, say that they feel worn-out and emotionally drained. At a time when everything should have been wonderful they are often exhausted from caring for a baby who is unsettled and difficult to manage. Parents need help and support to overcome these short-term crises of confidence. Some units have a liason health visitor or home care nurse to assist in this way and help reduce the problem of conflicting advice reported by so many mothers.

Different experiences

Parents who have had a premature baby have much in common, but not all of them experience the emotions and responses described here. The way in which they react to their baby being born too soon, and the events that follow, will depend on many different factors.

Mothers who have given birth by Caesarean section, particularly under general anaesthetic, find it harder to believe they have had a baby than those who gave birth normally. Women who have previously had an abortion can feel guilty that it may have contributed to the premature delivery of this baby. Like couples who have had one or more miscarriages before this live birth, they may be particularly disturbed and distressed by some aspects of the situation. These can include being in the same hospital, seeing the same staff, and being once more at the centre of medical attention.

Parents who have already had a preterm baby may again feel cheated and be intensely disappointed. But if their previous experience was favourable they may have more realistic expectations, and perhaps make a better adjustment over-all. For those who have given birth to a full-term baby before, a preterm birth can be even more of a shock. In this situation the new baby can present a depressing contrast, and unfavourable comparisons are only too easily made. Some parents feel more detached in these circumstances, finding it much harder to relate to their new very small baby, while others see him or her as something special and different.

Whatever the reaction, the conflict and difficulties for parents with other children at home should not be under-estimated. Alternative care arrangements may help, but are likely to give rise to yet more guilt and anxiety. On the other hand taking an older child to visit the neonatal unit can be stressful and so parents may find themselves uncertain about what to do.

Parents who have had twins may feel more overwhelmed, and feelings are further complicated when, as often happens, one baby is bigger or healthier than the other. If one baby dies, as with other multiple births where not all the infants do well, feelings towards the remaining baby can be very mixed. Mourning for one baby is always very difficult while caring for another (see p. 207).

The way in which parents react and try to come to terms with the preterm birth of their baby can be greatly affected by their own social circumstances. Single mothers, without a partner to share the worries and enjoy the baby's progress may feel extremely isolated unless they have a supportive family nearby. Problems of housing and unemployment can make the birth of a small, sick, baby seem like 'the last straw'. At this time the sensitive and positive help of a network of family and friends, and of professionals from the hospital and the community, can do much to turn what may seem like another failure into a success.

The reactions of relatives and friends

Relatives and friends anticipate the arrival of a new baby with much excitement. Once they are aware of the early birth their feelings parallel those of the parents. They are sad and sympathetic when the baby is ill, and feel elated when he begins to get better. But there may be other reactions too. Grandparents in particular usually feel an overwhelming desire to protect their own children from the pain and anguish they are going through, and to give them hope. Sometimes this may result in their being 'too interfering', or not giving the baby's parents 'room to breathe', when in fact they are trying so hard to be supportive. At the same time as they are wishing fervently for the baby's survival they may remember that 'in their day' such small babies often suffered severe handicap, and unwittingly convey a feeling of pessimism that conflicts with the doctors' outlook and what the parents have been told.

Friends with young children of their own may 'withdraw' during the crisis because they do not know how to respond. They may feel that the couple would prefer not to have painful reminders of families with healthy, 'normal' children. They may be unable to find comforting words to use, and have little idea of what goes on in a neonatal unit; this may prevent them from feeling comfortable in their conversations with the baby's parents and family.

Parents find it difficult and upsetting to explain the situation to relatives and neighbours. Inadvertent and thoughtless remarks at this time may hurt or alienate parents from the very people who could be giving them support. What is more useful is for them to let parents talk and to listen to what they have to say without brushing aside their fears or giving lots of advice.

There are times when parents wish they didn't have so many people ringing up for 'any news': the telephone may always seem to ring just as they're sitting down to eat, or about to rush off to the hospital. It should be remembered that a phone ringing causes panic for parents whose baby is ill. For this reason some families find it better to tell friends that they will get in touch instead, or to delegate this responsibility to another person. Practical help can be more useful than just calling to visit, and parents should not hesitate to ask friends if they would mind doing some shopping, looking after the children for a few hours, or preparing a simple supper. It may take courage to ring people up for favours, but families who have used their friends like this in times of crisis invariably report that their friendships are richer and stronger for the experience.

Parents' groups

In some neonatal units staff have encouraged the development of self-help groups for parents. In others parents themselves have taken an active role in this. The understanding and support that parents in similar situations can give to one another are of tremendous value, both when a baby is first born, and later on. The involvement of 'veteran' parents who have survived the anxious early months provides concrete proof that preterm babies do get better and grow well, and that their parents do manage to cope somehow.

Talking with other parents about practical problems, the shared experience of visiting a baby in hospital, and the worries about equipment or treatment, contributes positively to the well-being of the whole family. Many parents express the feeling that 'only another mother or father in the same situation could really understand'; this is an indication of the need for parents of preterm babies to be able to get together. Discussing their baby and their feelings on an equal footing and in a reciprocal way, in contrast to the unequal relationships that parents have with the doctors and nurses caring for their baby, can be of great benefit in helping them to come to terms with what has happened.

Sometimes a social worker or an experienced counsellor may be involved in setting up or running a parents' group. However their role is not one of an active participant but rather one of encouraging parents to come and talk.

There are local and national organisations, such as those concerned with the welfare of children in hospital, the problems of coping with twins, and various aspects of pregnancy and parenthood. These can provide help and information for parents of preterm babies, and are listed in the appendix.

The future

Anxiety about the long-term future and consequences of being born too soon concerns parents for a long time to come. They worry about the effects of the experience on the baby, and of the effect of the separation on themselves and their relationship with their child. The traumatic nature of the crises they went through is not easily forgotten, but though this period may be looked back on with sadness parents will remember the high points as their baby's health improved and he or she began to respond to them individually.

The long-term impact of a preterm birth on a family is difficult to gauge. The stresses and strains it can place on a couple's relationship are marked, and though many marriages survive intact some do not. Both parents may find that they are more emotional for quite some time: crying easily, losing their tempers more frequently, and generally being more irritable.

Feelings of anxiety and panic may continue to occur for some months. These usually fade in intensity unless a baby develops other medical problems or surgery is necessary. Readmission to hospital can bring back all the feelings of uncertainty experienced earlier, even when the baby's current problems are minor. Though parents do feel 'low' at times, very few become so depressed that they need treatment for their condition.

It is difficult to know whether these reactions might have occurred after the birth of a healthy full-term baby. Some may simply be part of the process of readjustment to life after the birth of a new baby, with disturbed nights, disorganized mealtimes, and less time for parents to spend together. Though the attitudes and feelings of parents are inevitably coloured by the fact that their baby was born too soon, they should avoid interpreting all aspects of his behaviour as being a consequence of his prematurity.

In the long term, fears about the baby's health and development, and worries about the effects of his being born too soon, continue to preoccupy parents for sometime. The vivid memories that many parents have of the experience, even years later, attest to the intensity of their feelings at the time.

Some special concerns about preterm twins

How do I keep from loving one more than the other?

Studies have shown that most parents develop a special affection for one of their preterm twins, although they may not feel able to admit to it. Some prefer the healthier baby, while others invest more time and emotion in the twin that is less healthy. Often an individual's preferences fluctuate and parents should not feel guilty about the way they 'distribute' their love. In time they come to find the right balance of affection and attention to meet the needs of both.

Will they be ready to go home together?

The progress of twins is never identical; even if their medical problems are similar, one may be quicker to gain weight or learn to feed than the other. However many hospitals have a policy of discharging both babies together. This is to lessen the chance of parents' developing excessively discrepant affection for the healthier one; it also obviates the problems of coping with a new set of demands at home while still travelling in to care for the baby in hospital. If one of your twins requires a much longer stay in hospital, perhaps because of surgery, it can seem particularly unfair to be deprived of both babies. Taking one home first can give you the opportunity to establish some routines and gain confidence. It is still possible to make the time spent with your sicker baby special so that she will fit into the family on coming home.

How will I ever cope with two preterm babies when I get home?

The first weeks at home with any twins are almost always exhausting so do not be too quick to blame your tiredness on the fact that they were preterm or on their 'Special Care' experience. The best preparation is probably several nights rooming in on a postnatal ward or neonatal unit so that you get to know each baby's pattern of feeding and sleeping over continuous 24-hour periods. Once home practical support from your partner is invaluable, as is a paid domestic help if you can afford it. A supportive health visitor, community nurse, and other parents of twins can also offer advice and encouragement.

Will they develop at the same rate after birth?

When a baby is very preterm or sick his early behaviour, growth, and development is likely to be most influenced by his medical problems. So even when twins are genetically 'identical', if, for example, one has been on a ventilator for many weeks he may take longer to learn to feed and to become alert and interested in his surroundings. And if one of them has grown poorly *in utero* from early on in the pregnancy, then his weight and length may continue to differ from those of his sibling. These differences serve to emphasize each baby's uniqueness, and differences in personality are frequently apparent also.

One of my twins is so sick I don't think she'll survive. Is it very wrong to spend more time with her brother?

When only one twin is critically ill, there is sometimes a reluctance to become too 'attached' to the sick one. But your baby's condition may not be as hopeless as it seems, and even if she dies, then having the memories of being with her to look back on usually brings an inner peace and the consolation that you were able to love and care for her even though she lived for only a brief time. After a serious illness and much uncertainty, there is often a sense of relief when a baby dies; you should try not to feel guilty that this turning point frees you to spend all your time with her twin. It can take a long while to get over the contradiction of losing half of a pregnancy while still needing to care for and enjoy the other half.

You will probably always continue to think of your son as a twin, but as your grief lessens over the months, you will be able to strengthen your relationship with him while still cherishing the memories of his sister.

10

The needs of
other children
in the family

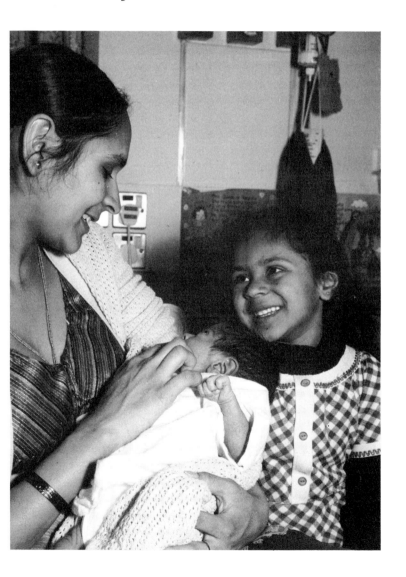

A new arrival

Any child feels threatened to some extent by the birth of a new baby. This is particularly so when he is an only child; the focus of everyone's attention is suddenly changed, and he is displaced from the centre of things. His needs, routines, territory, and even belongings, come to be of secondary importance compared with the more immediate demands of a newer, smaller, arrival, who seems to do nothing but sleep or cry. Many studies have shown that the age and personality of the child, his degree of preparedness for the new baby, and the sensitivity of his parents to his feelings, all affect his adjustment to the new baby.

For the children of those few mothers who have needed a prolonged stay in hospital before the birth of a preterm baby, there may have been opportunities to become familiar with the hospital environment. Although preparation may prevent some of the emotional disturbances described later in this chapter, their father may be the only person who can provide the stability and sympathy required by them at this time.

After the birth of a preterm or ill baby there are a number of events which may frighten or disturb children who are too young to put their feelings into words. Even a young toddler needs to be told about the unexpected birth. Because it was early neither parents nor children will have had time to make practical or emotional preparations. The threatened birth often presents a crisis which may involve an ambulance, hurried telephone calls, and leaving the children suddenly with a friend, or relation. These events may be followed by a long antenatal stay in hospital before their mother shows any sign of producing the awaited brother or sister. After having the baby a mother may also have to stay longer than originally anticipated. This may be because of a Caesarean section, her high blood pressure, or an infection.

In the early days parents can be very upset and worried about the new baby's chances of survival; their mood swings and feelings of sadness, anger, or impatience, and sometimes overprotective behaviour, are difficult for children to understand. When parents are away visiting the baby for much of the day for what can be weeks on end, the children lose their company and emotional availability without the compensating pleasure and pride of helping to care for the new baby. Even when a child is taken along to visit he may become bored with the limited activities available in a hospital, and resent these daily outings which interfere with normal routines, and seem to take precedence over his own wishes.

Although evidence suggests that it is beneficial for children to visit the neonatal unit, hospitals can certainly seem like frightening places. This is especially so if a child has previously visited grandparents, or very ill relatives, who have subsequently died. The sight of needles, wires, blood, tubes, and white coats, may lead a child to believe that doctors and nurses are hurting rather than helping their new brother or sister. To a young child it may even appear that the baby is 'tied up', or 'put in a plastic box without any air'. These thoughts are not ones that children bring out easily for fear of having them dismissed as being 'silly', or in case it results in exclusion from visits.

Children of pre-school age may imagine that all actions and events going on around them are somehow related to themselves and so a child may feel responsible for the sickness of the new baby. He can feel it is his 'badness' in not wanting the baby enough, or telling a lie, or failing to finish his dinner, which has caused all the pain for the baby and has hurt the parents he really loves. In this way a young child may feel that the baby is being punished for something that he himself did wrong, and in turn may expect to be punished.

In this situation a child is often uncharacteristically very good, or deliberately naughty, to test his parents and see whether they still love him. He might also imagine that if life is so fragile that a new baby becomes sick then he too might die soon. Some children who happen to see the baby asleep, having seen him awake and moving before, may think that the baby has died. In a young child there may be a nagging doubt that if his parents were really satisfied with him they would not have wanted another baby at all. Thus a child may invent ways of getting rid of the baby and later feel guilty about such 'bad' thoughts.

All these hidden anxieties are shown in individual ways but the most common effect is that the child reverts to more immature habits and to old comforts. He may start wetting his pants, wetting the bed, wanting a bottle, a dummy, or a feed at the breast. He may demand old toys or comforters that had been put away. He may simply sulk or become moody, have temper tantrums, or deliberately try to provoke his parents, brothers and sisters, or the new baby. These are all signs that a child needs extra reassurance and sympathy rather than any punishment.

Making things easier

Nothing can totally erase the feeling of deprivation and upset that children have who suddenly find that their parents are hardly ever at home. When they are at home parents may be so completely preoccupied or weepy that they 'aren't fun any more'. Armed with an understanding of what these events can mean to a child, and some careful thought and planning, parents can do a great deal to help their children to adapt to the situation brought about by the preterm birth of a brother or sister. These efforts should aim at lessening the emotional burden placed on the children, trying to minimize the disruption to their usual routines, and maintaining a sense of family.

Lessening the emotional burden

One of the big problems that parents with one or more other children have is trying to keep a balance between their own grief and anxiety, and the need to present a calm front to avoid causing any upsets.

Young children generally expect certain things of adults: that they are in control, that they can be trusted, and that they can 'make it better' when things are not going well. During the crisis of preterm birth the behaviour of adults is unpredictable. Parents have the difficult task of helping their children understand that their baby brother or sister is sick, or small, but that the doctors and nurses are helping him to get better, and that with time the baby will be like other new babies. This is especially hard for parents when they themselves may be in doubt about the outcome. They need to explain that a baby who arrived too soon has to grow a bit more in hospital, and that as this takes place their own feelings of sadness and anger will gradually disappear.

Parents should emphasize to the child at home that he is still precious to them, despite their obvious preoccupation with the new baby. They can make it easier by showing some of their distress while explaining that even 'grown-ups' need to cry sometimes. It is better to acknowledge to a child who has some understanding of these emotions that this is how the parents are feeling. To most children it is quite clear when parents are upset or unhappy without them actually having to say so. The strain of presenting a positive and happy picture of all being well is an extra burden which parents at this time could well do without. Short outbursts of real feelings are preferable to pretence, though reassurance is needed after such episodes; following these with a cuddle and a game (even for older children) will do much to restore the normal equilibrium.

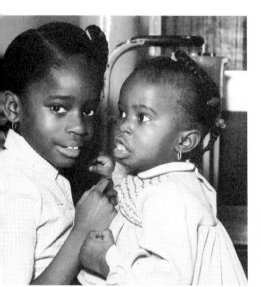 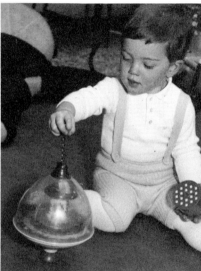

Older brothers or sisters can often keep a younger one entertained during a hospital visit; however, having safe and appropriate toys around is essential.

For the children who visit the baby unit it is important that those who are old enough be introduced to the staff and have some of the equipment and procedures explained simply to them. Some of their fears can be minimized, or even prevented, in this way. They may be helped to accept the strange and unusual environment of the neonatal unit as a friendly one in which the newest member of the family is being looked after for the time being.

Minimizing disruption to routines

Daily routines can be extremely important for children, particularly the under-fives, and if at all possible visits to the hospital should be scheduled so as *not* to coincide with the most important of these. For younger children there are often special rituals that maximize co-operation at bed, bath, or meal-times; examples of these are 'flying' the spoon to his mouth with aeroplane noises, tickling him in a certain way while saying a familiar rhyme, or finding the right toy or blanket that can be held whilst falling asleep.

A toddler is very aware of changes in the behaviour of those taking care of him, but with little or no language skills he is essentially non-verbal and thus cannot remind his parents that they aren't doing things in the usual way. Parents need to stop and think in the rush to get out of the door in the evening, or as they worry about the new baby, about whether they are providing the familiar routines for him each day. In order to make sure that a substitute care-giver, even Dad, knows about all the 'little' things that make up a small child's day it is best to have him or her go through an entire day with the mother, rather than just being told of the schedule of events, or given a list. Even small changes can greatly add to the trauma and heighten the pain of separation.

The improved verbal ability of pre-school children enables them to tell the person looking after them what actually needs to be done; about favourite foods, stories that are told at bedtime, and games that are usually played. They may assert their feelings of independence by wanting to do everything for themselves, or alternatively revert to more babyish habits. Either can be very trying for those looking after them. An established pattern of regular attendance at a play-group or nursery school can do a great deal to maintain some order and continuity in the lives of children who are not yet at full-time school.

The school-age child tends to have a life outside the family which satisfies some of his needs for social status, feelings of importance, and achievement. Routines for him may be more a question of responsibilities than 'perks'. It can be difficult for parents to know whether reduced co-operation is a genuine reaction to stress, or a skilful attempt to avoid homework, or other not so pleasant household chores. Tact and recognition that even a 10 or 12 year old may feel some conflict over the new baby and be disturbed by parents' anxious behaviour, can go a long way towards avoiding confrontation. Although an older child is generally quite capable of remembering regular events like 'Cubs' or 'Brownies', or important occasions such as sports days or birthday parties, with all that is going on even these may be forgotten. Parents must also be careful not to forget the other things that are important like pocket-money, or making time to shop for a birthday present.

Maintaining a sense of family

In their determination to do what is best for the new baby parents often bend over backwards to visit the neonatal unit at every opportunity. They may visit together for most of the time because of the travelling convenience and mutual support. But unless such visits take place after the other children are asleep daily hospital visits which exclude brothers and sisters reinforce the fact that life for them is now quite different.

After weeks of this it may seem to a young child that his world will never return to normal. At this time parents do need to emphasize that such disruptions are only short-term and will not go on forever. A new baby in the family does bring about many changes, but the immediate anxieties that are to do with his being in hospital will pass and life will settle down, although it will never be quite the same again. It is worth making an effort to see that some family activities are preserved; having at least one meal a day together, making time for a game or two in the evening, or going shopping as a family, may help. Sometimes changing the pattern of visiting so that each parent goes to see the new baby separately, is the only solution when a pre-school child's behaviour indicates that he or she is acutely missing their company.

Perhaps the most important way of generating a 'family' feeling is by involving the other children with the new baby as soon as is practical. If possible they should visit the new baby so that they can see for themselves what he looks like, where he is, and who is taking care of him.

A good way of maintaining their interest during the hospital stay is to keep a scrap-book of the baby and his progress. Photographs can be taken in the neonatal unit of the child next to the incubator and of him giving the small brother or sister a toy. Later on he may be given the opportunity to hold the baby. These photographs, together with the usual pictures of the baby, and the drawings that the child may have made showing changes in what is happening to the baby, can be put in the book. 'Souvenirs' of his treatment, for example an empty syringe, a feeding tube, phototherapy mask, or bottle teat, can be incorporated. This kind of activity serves a number of purposes. Firstly it helps children appreciate the fact that the baby is growing and making progress by highlighting the small changes that they might not otherwise notice. It also gives them, and the rest of the family, a way of looking back through the baby's first year and provides a means of putting that part of the baby's and family's life into perspective.

Talking to the child about what he draws may help parents to be certain that he is not misinterpreting what is going on, particularly in relation to the medical procedures that he may have seen. For an older child such a book is useful in that it can be shown to class-mates at school, proving that there really is a new baby in the family. At the same time it provides a useful basis for classroom discussions on birth, growth, differences between individuals, and what goes on in hospitals or within families.

Play is an excellent activity in which children 'act out' some of their worries and fears. Toy medical kits, and an adapted shoe box 'incubator' with a baby-like doll and sticky tape, can provide a basis for going over some of the things they may have seen happen to babies on the unit. Play also provides parents with insight into their children's perception of what is happening in the hospital, and may enable the child to come to terms with the disruption to his life and the changed family dynamics.

A younger child can be given rather simpler tasks which underline his importance at home, such as helping to get things ready for the new baby. As a morning or evening ritual the new baby's things could be arranged, and any new toys placed in the waiting cot or crib. Because a young child's sense of time is poor he needs tangible proof that the days are passing. Ticking off the days on a big calendar, collecting a stone or leaf each day for the baby, or making pictures to decorate the wall near the baby's cot, emphasize the passing of time. Although such activities can be time-consuming and difficult for parents to maintain over a long period, they make their other children more aware of family ties, of notions of 'belonging', and of the importance of their own role in making preparations for the new baby.

If an older child chooses a present for the baby, such as a small soft toy of the sort described in Chapter 6, it can be seen at each visit, and as the baby matures and becomes more alert the child may actually see him looking at the present. Sometimes parents buy a toy for an older child and say it is a present from the baby, but unless the child is really quite young he is not likely to believe this story. Simply getting a present for an older child when the new baby arrives, and suggesting that relations and friends do the same if they wish, may help him feel less left out of all the excitement associated with the new baby's arrival.

Coping with changes in behaviour

It is a rare child who does not show some change in his mood, behaviour, or habits, when a new baby arrives. It is helpful for parents to make children of all ages aware of the fact that they know that their children may not be feeling the same as usual, and that they may be sad, angry, fed-up, or lonely, after what has happened. It is probably better to assume that any negative behaviours are a reflection of the present situation so that parents can approach the problem from that standpoint.

As previously mentioned, a premature birth can mean a crisis for the whole family. In this situation a child is likely to test or worry a parent more, and the parent may have to display more patience than usual. Telling parents that their child will 'get over it' in time may reassure them about the long term but they also need help with behavioural problems at a more practical level. A 'night-light' in the bedroom if a child has become frightened of the dark, or giving a recently toilet-trained child the chance of going back into nappies if things seem to be getting too much for him, are the kind of strategies that are worth trying. In offering a child these possibilities it is important for the parent to let him know that when he is a bit happier, and the household a little more settled, he can always give them up. Allowing a child to regress or go back a little, without teasing or recrimination, can reassure some children. This is particularly important to realize, since demands are frequently made of older children following the birth of a brother or sister that it is now time to grow up and do away with babyish habits. These expectations are not always spoken but none the less felt. Putting on pressure in this way, at a time when parents are worried and upset, is likely to result in conflict, and possibly more serious behaviour problems. The months after a new baby is taken home are when most older children show that they have indeed become more grown up by helping in the care and entertainment of the newest family member.

Giving an older child other responsibilities, like looking after and caring for a pet, can also help. Some families find it useful either to have a child take over some of the care of a family pet already with them, or to be responsible for choosing and looking after a new one. However this can be expensive and time-consuming; a new puppy or kitten at home is more than most parents in this situation can cope with! Thus if an animal is bought for this reason a pet that is relatively easy to care for is a more practical and sensible answer.

Children in stressful situations often sleep poorly, have nightmares, wake more at night, and wet their bed. With all these problems, although patience and reassurance are very important, talking to a child about the things bothering him may help him understand and resolve them. Other people, including teachers, need to be made aware of the situation. All must recognize that a child's own explanations of why he is behaving differently from normal may not be the same as his subconscious thoughts about what is happening in his world at this moment. It may be difficult to get through to the child at this time. Some months, or even years later on, discussions between parents and child may enable both to gain a better understanding of how they felt about the birth and hospitalization of their preterm baby.

In the short term, medication can help with some of these problems. It is often a useful way of breaking the pattern of nightwaking or bed-wetting that a child has got into, and provides a breathing space for both the child and his already over-burdened parents. Advice from the family doctor, or talking the problem over with the local health visitor, may be helpful. Alternatively parents may prefer to discuss things with the hospital paediatrician whom they already know.

Some children continue to sleep perfectly well but during the day may be more aggressive to parents or to other children. Others have full-blown temper tantrums or breath-holding attacks whenever they cannot have what they want. Others become more faddy about the foods they will eat, or the way meals are presented. These problems may have arisen before and are ways in which an anxious or stressed child shows his feelings. Depending on the child, and the parents' own views and experience, each family tries to deal with these problems in their own way. A strategy of preventing the child from hurting himself or others without punishing him, ignoring minor infringements of the rules, distracting him where possible, and not worrying if he only eats a narrow range of foods, is often the best answer. However parents with a sick or small preterm baby to worry about can over-react to what appears to be deliberately antisocial and provocative behaviour from an older child. From this a child can easily get the message that this new baby is even more special and more important than he is to his parents. At the same time it must be remembered that much of the way an older child behaves at the time of the preterm birth of a sibling is typical of many children when a new baby arrives, and is not peculiar to these circumstances.

A positive note

This chapter has necessarily described how the situation may appear from the point of view of the other children in the family. A great responsibility is placed on the shoulders of parents at a time when they themselves may be unhappy and anxious. It may be unreasonable to expect parents to be sympathetic and responsive at such a difficult time for them. However, other children who need to be cared for at home can be a great comfort and distraction for parents. Many have remarked that an older child has kept them going, cheered them up, and made them laugh at a time when they would not have thought it possible. Answering another child's needs, helping to keep their lives as normal as possible, and gaining extra emotional support from more cuddles and contact, has helped many parents come through this difficult period.

11

Ready to go home

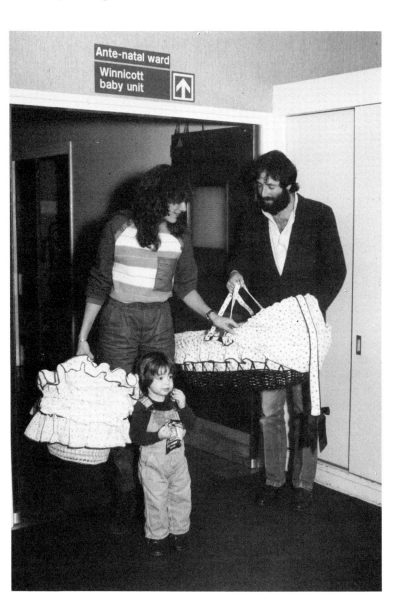

Taking a new baby home is a momentous occasion for any parent, and doubly precious when a baby has been in hospital for some time. If they had not previously decorated a room, or made or bought things for the baby before the birth, most parents of a preterm baby cannot bear to do so until they feel certain that there really will be a baby coming home with them.

The last week or so of care in hospital can seem intolerable to parents, especially when they see that their baby is growing well, is no longer sick, and only on minimal monitoring. Many find themselves imagining and 'rehearsing' this step long in advance, but at the same time they try not to think too much about it in case their hopes do not come true.

Hospital criteria for discharge

Most neonatal units do not now have a fixed policy for discharging babies from their care. Each baby's readiness to leave the hospital is decided by considering several different factors: whether he is feeding well, gaining weight steadily, and if there are no remaining medical problems that need hospital treatment. However, there are still a few units which specify that a baby must reach a certain weight, for example 2.3 kg (5 lb), before being taken home. In contrast to this some baby units may occasionally send babies home weighing as little as 1500 gm (3 lb 5 oz). As a rough guide one might expect a preterm baby to stay in hospital until he is near his expected date of delivery at term.

Reasons for delay

The most common reason for a delay in discharging a preterm baby is that he is not taking enough feed by himself. Premature babies usually begin on naso-gastric or naso-jejunal tube-feeds, and then progress to the breast, or bottle-feeds (see Chapter 7). They may take a long time to 'get the hang of it' and to learn to feed 'orally' in the normal way.

Parents often express feelings of disappointment and anger at their preterm baby for being slow and difficult in feeding. They may also be annoyed with, or irritated by, nursing staff for seeming inflexible with the feeding schedules, or for not being as patient or responsive to the baby's behaviour during feeds as they themselves might be.

If a mother is breast-feeding she may decide to give up in case her baby's lack of progress might result in extra days or weeks in hospital, even though this strategy is not likely to make any difference. Mothers need a great deal of support at this stage to help them accept the ups and downs in feeding, and they need to be told that progress may be very unexpected and sudden.

When a baby is almost ready for discharge it is most important to give parents some warning. Even the good news that a baby is finally ready to go home can be overwhelming and can cause feelings of panic. Everyone needs the opportunity to respond to this challenge in their own way and in their own time.

At this stage many parents feel torn between trying to visit their baby as much as possible, and in getting everything ready at home. In spite of the rush and worry of last minute shopping, decorating, and even house-moving, they do cope when the time comes.

Living-in with the baby before going home

Where hospitals have the resources it is becoming increasingly common to offer the mother the chance to stay and share the same room as her baby for one or two days before the baby is discharged home. This allows her to gain experience in having full responsibility for the baby's care on a 24 hour basis, but with support and advice available if needed. Sometimes there are facilities for the father to stay too.

This 'rooming-in' can take many different forms. The mother

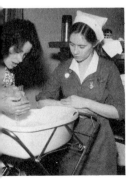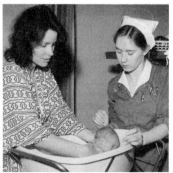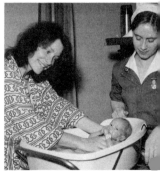

Bathing their preterm baby alarms many mothers, so helpful guidance is particularly welcome during the 'rooming-in' period.

may be admitted to a postnatal ward with other mothers and their newborn infants, or to a single room nearby. Some hospitals have one or more rooms that are adjacent to the neonatal unit and are available for this specific purpose. In hospitals which have a 'transitional care' ward for infants needing extra medical care or supervision, the mother may be admitted there. A few units in the United States have devised a system whereby mothers and babies are able to stay together for several weeks if necessary in a special self-contained apartment unit.

Whatever system is in operation many parents are grateful that they can be together with their baby within the hospital environment. 'I knew that if I needed it help was near', 'We bathed him together on our own for the first time—it was great!', 'Staying in the hospital for a couple of days gave me a chance to be alone with my baby and get to know him better without the other children around'.

Although many mothers are grateful for this opportunity to become more confident in handling their baby, it is obviously not practical or desirable for all. If there are other young children at home, or where arrangements for school-age children mean that the father has to take time off work it is usually necessary for the mother to be back at home as soon as possible. If she is going to have trained professional help at home (such as a nanny or a nurse) a mother may feel that a hospital stay is unnecessary. Most mothers do not welcome a return to hospital food and routines, even for a few days, though many are willing to put up with them for the sake of the baby if encouraged to do so.

It is essential that liaison between the neonatal unit and the postnatal ward is maintained to ensure that 'rooming in' is a good and positive experience for mothers. Women having their first baby, and lacking previous experience, and all mothers with pre-term babies, are very vulnerable and need consistent rather than conflicting advice. Nothing is more disheartening on the last night in hospital than to be told, or have it inferred, that 'what you are doing is all wrong' and that the feeding, changing and bathing routines that you have worked out should be done differently. At this stage confidence-building is important for parents who have had a small or sick baby born too soon; this is the time when they and their baby will have to begin to manage without all the technical equipment and skilled care that has been available up to now.

The responsibility can seem immense, even to those parents who have managed to recover their self-confidence after the shattering experience of having a preterm baby.

Sensitive and perceptive staff can help enormously at this point, but it requires considerable tact and self-control to provide support for parents while at the same time managing not to interfere with the ways in which they, as responsible adults, have chosen to care for their baby.

Medicines and reminders at discharge

In the excitement of getting ready to take the baby home it is easy to forget instructions about medicines and vitamins to be given at home. Many neonatal units give a 'discharge sheet' on which is described the type and amount of feed the baby has been taking, his current weight, and a detailed list of the medications to be given; the amount, how often they should be given, and whether they can be combined or not, may be stated (Table 11.1). Future hospital appointments may also be listed there. Parents need to know why follow-up appointments are made so that they do not then mistakenly believe that their baby is to be brought back to the hospital because he is still ill, or because he necessarily has problems or a potential handicap. Though a baby may be seen by the family doctor and be regularly attending the local health clinic, specialist follow-ups are valuable both to the medical staff caring for preterm babies, and to parents whose baby was hospitalized for some time (Chapter 13). Parents often feel reassured at the prospect of future appointments with a doctor who cared for their baby when he was small, and whom they met several times in the neonatal unit.

Going home at last

Towards the end of a baby's stay in hospital parents are usually encouraged to take over as much of the baby's care as possible. However, actually taking their baby home represents a very real and tangible transfer of responsibility from the hospital to the parents. Within the hospital environment they have probably been quite sheltered, and to varying degrees institutionalized, but now all the decisions are up to them. Taking their preterm baby home and becoming a normal family again is for many parents an enormous step. It is often accompanied by a mixture of excitement and trepidation, and may be pervaded by a sense of unreality: 'I could hardly believe the time had come at last', 'When you want something so much you worry it may never happen', 'I couldn't wait to dress him and take him home, but at the same time I was worried about whether I could manage'.

The first few days at home for many parents is a 'honeymoon' period. Despite the endless round of nappies, feeds, and checks to see if their baby is all right, many parents feel elated. 'It was wonderful to have her with us and to be able to feed her comfortably in our own bed', 'At last I can have my baby completely to myself', 'When he was in hospital and I was at home it was like part of me was missing, now we are a complete family'. However, as with the birth of any new baby the excitement gradually fades, life changes, adjustments are made, and though often tired and sometimes worried most parents would say 'We wouldn't be without him for the world'.

Now that your baby is going home here are some things that you might want to refer to:

Table 11.1

Last recorded weight   _____ grams   (_____ lb _____ oz)

Suggested feeding

Breast
How often? Just whenever your baby seems hungry.

Bottle
How often? As often as he/she seems hungry but at least _____ hourly (_____ feeds per day). Formula—(brand...............) _____ scoops to _____ ml (_____ oz) cooled boiled water. How much? Offer _____ ml (_____ oz) each feed and if your baby finishes the bottle every time put a little extra volume in for future feeds. Do not expect your baby always to finish the bottle. REMEMBER TO MEASURE FORMULA FEEDS ACCURATELY.

Medicines (Vitamins, Iron, Antibiotics, etc.)

	Name	Volume	Number of doses per day
1.	_____	_____	_____
2.	_____	_____	_____
3.	_____	_____	_____
4.	_____	_____	_____

Any special instructions:_____

Appointments at follow-up clinic

	Date	Time	Place
1.	_____	_____	_____
2.	_____	_____	_____

Reasons for seeking medical advice for your baby

1. If you notice a sudden change in his/her behaviour e.g. if your baby becomes lethargic or disinterested in feeds.
2. If your baby starts vomiting more than usual or develops diarrhoea.
3. If he/she seems feverish.

If you are worried or have any questions your family doctor should be able to help you; alternatively you may always bring your baby to the Casualty Department at .... Hospital or get advice by telephoning us (Tel. ....)

Health visitor

Name: _____ *Clinic:* _____ *Tel. no:* _____

12

The early weeks
at home

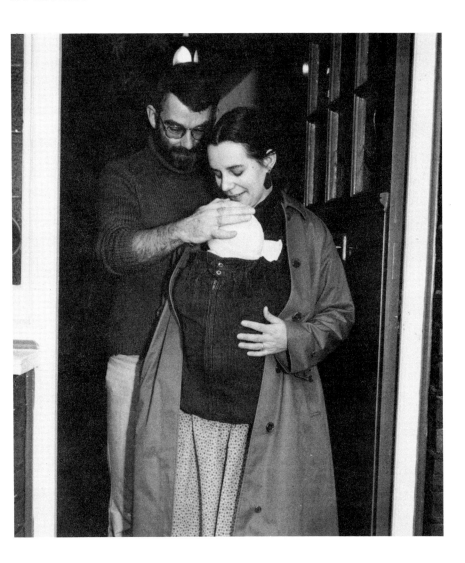

Practical concerns

Many parents with a new baby will have bought, or been given, one or two practical books on babycare which cover development, common problems, and illnesses. However, no matter how much your preterm baby has grown, and how healthy he is pronounced to be by the medical staff, he may still seem less robust and quite vulnerable to you. It is entirely natural, therefore, to worry about how you will manage without the reassurance that comes from apnoea alarms, warm nurseries, and regular weighing and temperature checks. With any loss of confidence in their own role as parents, and without the round the clock advice and support of qualified medical staff, it is easy to feel uncertain about what seem to be routine and trivial questions such as 'Is the bedroom warm enough?' But at the back of many parents' minds may be the more important question 'What shall we do if something goes wrong?'

The situation is often made more difficult by conflicting advice that may descend on you the moment you are ready to take the baby home! Friends and relations can be enormously supportive over the early months but few are likely to know how preterm babies respond and behave. The health visitor and family doctor are good sources of advice about child health care and development but occasionally they too may forget that a baby's age should be 'corrected' for his early birth when evaluating his development. It may not occur to them that parents will have more questions than usual because of the stressful time they have come through, and that some parents continue to be anxious for the first year or so.

Although a preterm baby needs care similar to that of any other baby coming home, parents may worry more because of his smaller size and the problems he had when younger. There are also a few ways in which his growth and health problems may differ from the full-term newborn. The following section is a collection of the most common questions asked by parents in the first few months after their preterm baby has been discharged. Increasing knowledge and experience will enable you to come to know what is normal and right for your own baby, and to recognize when to seek professional advice.

What will I need to have at home?

Most baby books give a basic list of clothes needed for the new-born, and the requirements of the preterm infant are little different. However a common worry for most parents is where to find clothes and nappies (diapers) small enough for the baby going home weighing less than the typical 3.6 kg (7 lb 14 oz) newborn. European manufacturers of baby clothes have long produced size 54 and 56 cm garments, in contrast to the standard UK size 60, but these can be expensive. More recently a specialist manufacturer of dolls' clothes came up with the idea of making small garments for small babies, and some national chainstores now produce 'thermal' ranges of preterm clothing. 'Parentcraft' magazines are a good source of information about new products.

Properly fitting nappies may be hard to find, even though several manufacturers produce preterm sizes for hospital use. Some chemists (drugstores) are willing to place a regular order, or the hospital staff may be able to suggest an address to write to. Alternatively the smallest pads can be used with cut-down plastic tie-pants, or the disposable pads that can be purchased in a roll can be cut to size. Mothers using cloth nappies cut them in half, or use triangular shapes which have less bulk around the leg.

Within a few months your baby will have grown into 'first size' clothes and nappies. Before this, many mothers prefer to dress their baby in the smaller sizes which are more flattering and do not simply exaggerate their baby's smallness. It is best not to buy too many very small garments because preterm babies can grow rather fast!

Feeding

If my baby is bottle-fed, how much should be offered at each bottle feed?

Most neonatal units will note down how much the baby has been taking in the days before he is ready for home. It is unusual for a baby to take exactly the same amount of milk each time—just like adults, sometimes he will feel like having a snack, and at others a large meal. It may take a while to learn the length of time that he normally takes to finish a bottle.

It is a good idea to put a little more milk in his bottle than he is expected to finish, but always throw away what is left. In this way he will continue to have sufficient milk for his growth needs as he gets bigger and as his demands increase.

As a rough guide he is likely to consume between 150 and 210 ml (5–7 oz) per kg of body weight during each 24 hours. For example, a baby who weighs 3 kg, and who is having 5 feeds over 24 hours, should be drinking between 90 and 125 ml (3–4 oz) each feed.

What type of milk is best for him?

If the neonatal unit has been happy with his weight gain it is better to leave him on the milk he is used to unless you are advised otherwise. However, there is very little difference between the specially adapted baby formula feeds. Ordinary cows milk (i.e. 'doorstep' milk, supermarket milk) is *not* suitable for babies until they are at least 8–12 months after their expected date of delivery. Even then the GP or paediatrician may have reasons for keeping a baby on formula milk for longer, so any changes should be discussed with him first.

Bottle-fed babies may occasionally need a bottle of plain boiled water, but this is unnecessary for a breast-fed baby unless the weather is particularly hot, or if he is feverish. When he is 3 months past his expected date of delivery your baby may be offered dilute fruit juice, such as orange or blackcurrant juice. Water used to mix these drinks should be boiled, and extra sugar should not be added.

How do I know if he's getting enough?

If a baby seems contented, and isn't crying out regularly in less than 2 hours, then he's having enough for his needs. Even if he is fussing a great deal hunger is not the only possible reason for this. The presence or absence of normal weight-gain recorded at a child health clinic, or by your doctor, may help to determine whether he is really underfed. A breast-feeding mother who is concerned about whether her baby is getting enough should offer the breast more frequently and let her baby nurse for longer.

Can a preterm baby get too fat?

It is unusual for babies who have been born early to become too fat on formula or breast-feeding. However, if he has had serious breathing problems in the first few weeks of life it is advisable to try to prevent him from becoming overweight since excess fatness seems to predispose to further periods of chestiness over the first year. Excess weight gain is more likely to occur when a baby is weaned on to solids at about 5-6 months; this is discussed in greater detail in the question about 'solids'.

Why does he make noises when he feeds?

Babies often gulp their feeds and this is a noisy process; grunts and splutters are the norm. Should a baby develop a snuffle (see p. 179) he is likely to have difficulty feeding, and if he appears to start coughing during the feed he should be allowed to take a break. Many people have commented that the preterm infant seems to make a particular soft snorting noise at times, particularly when feeding; this may be due to floppiness of the soft part of the palate which then vibrates causing the sound. Hiccups too are common in preterm babies and are a normal phenomenon.

Although breathlessness during feeds is rare, any parent who is concerned about their baby's breathing patterns should see a doctor for an explanation. 'Noises' are one of the ways that a young baby has of communicating, and although some babies are easily distracted during their bursts of sucking they may respond to being talked to during winding or at the end of the feed.

When will I be able to stop supplementing the breast-feeds with formula?

Some of you will still be offering formula-feeds as well as the breast when your baby comes home. You should make certain that you always offer formula *after a feed*, not before, so that your baby does not fill up on the formula first. You will find that as you breast-feed more often the amount of milk you produce usually starts to increase. You may notice that your baby begins to take less and less of the formula 'top-up' that you offer until it is eventually unnecessary. If this does not happen then try cutting back the formula by half the amount while allowing him to suckle longer at each feed. Then gradually reduce the top-up until he is fully breast-fed.

In spite of trying these tactics a number of mothers of preterm infants report that they were never able to cut out the formula supplement without the baby crying a lot, or failing to put on weight. Breast-feeding with a formula supplement (for some or all of the feeds) is a perfectly acceptable way to continue feeding a baby, and provides a feeling of closeness and fulfilment that some mothers feel they would forfeit by changing completely to bottle-feeding.

What should I do if I think my milk is drying up?

The more often you give your baby the chance to breast-feed the more milk you will produce. Try increasing the frequency with which your baby is offered the breast (perhaps every two hours for a day or so). Particularly after the anxious weeks in hospital, and the rather exhausing ones that follow homecoming, it may take a while for your milk flow to adjust to the baby's demands. Make sure that you are drinking plenty of fluids and eating a well-balanced diet with high protein foods (such as meat, fish, eggs, and cheese) rather than exclusively relying on cakes and chocolate bars. It is essential for a mother to set aside time for more rest if her milk supply seems to be diminishing; household tasks must take second place.

Many mothers find that expressing milk after feeds leads to a better milk supply by ensuring that her breasts are emptied each time. This expressed milk can be frozen for use at other times. Often, once breast-feeding is established, a mother's body has adjusted so well that her breasts no longer feel overly full and her let-down reflex is not so pronounced. This can lead to her thinking that her milk supply is failing. When she doubts her ability to produce enough milk, expressing after each feed for a few days can provide proof that milk is really available to meet her baby's needs. Some mothers 'drip' breast milk from the opposite breast to that from which the baby is suckling and this provides further evidence that they are secreting milk. Postnatal and breast-feeding support groups can be a great help when breast-feeding problems occur (see Appendix 2, p. 231).

What should I do if my baby refuses a feed?

Most babies at some time or another refuse a feed. If your baby appears normally alert and healthy this shouldn't worry you. If at the time when he would have been due for the next feed he continues to be disinterested or apathetic then you should seek medical advice. Of course there will come a time when your baby sleeps right through the night, and that is a bonus to look forward to!

Are my baby's stools normal?

The stools (motions) of fully breast-fed babies are usually more loose than those of formula-fed infants, and may be quite 'watery'. They can vary according to the food a mother is having. Stool colour is affected by bile pigments, and by some of the supplements, such as iron, that your baby may be receiving. The colour may change from day to day, being bright yellow, green, or dark. Alterations in consistency and odour often occur in relation to dietary changes. It is the changes in consistency occurring in the absence of an obvious dietary explanation—becoming very hard, or more loose and frequent—for which you may need to seek medical advice.

When should a preterm baby start on solid foods?

Opinions and fashions about giving solid foods change frequently, even for full-term infants. However, in view of the relative immaturity of the preterm baby's digestive system it is best to delay introducing solids until about 5 months after the expected date of delivery. You should ignore remarks about 'feeding up' your preterm baby because he was smaller at birth.

The general trend in infant feeding is toward the exclusion of 'gluten' (wheat, rye, barley, and oats) in the early months. Almost all commercial ranges include a number of 'gluten-free' flavours in their single and mixed foods which are marked with an international symbol. For this reason rice-based cereals are preferable to wheat and rusk types, at the beginning. When solid foods are introduced it is better to begin with sieved or blended chicken, vegetables, or stewed fruit. Babies need a week or so to get used to a new taste and this enables you to evaluate whether a new food suits him. It also takes a while for a baby to get used to the different tongue action involved in taking food from a spoon; early on he may spit out almost as much as goes in.

If there is an allergic predisposition ('atopy') in the family it is worth being extra careful when introducing solids. A few foods seem to cause more allergic reactions than others: dairy products (milk, butter, cheese, yoghurt), eggs, fish, 'pipped' fruits (oranges, apples, grapes, etc.), and wheat-based bread and cereals. There are plenty of alternatives to these on the market, and proprietary brands should be examined carefully to see if these particular ingredients are included on the label. Radical changes or omissions from the baby's diet can lead to deficiencies of certain nutrients, so any marked alterations are best discussed with your health visitor, doctor, or staff at the hospital clinic. Vegetarian diets are quite healthy for preterm babies too, but it is important to include milk. Some doctors might consider that babies on a vegetarian diet should remain on formula milk, rather than changing to ordinary milk delivered to the door or bought in the supermarket.

Keeping warm

How warm should my home be?

A temperature that is comfortable for an adult in shirt sleeves or a blouse will be warm enough for a 2 kg (4 lb 4 oz) baby going home. A minimum of 68 °F (20 °C) should be aimed at. It is draughts and fluctuations in room temperature—coldness at night or at bath times—that small babies have difficulty compensating for. This is not meant to imply that every room needs to be specially warmed, but the room he spends most time in should be kept at an even, comfortable temperature.

How should he be dressed to go out?

You will soon learn to judge if your baby is too hot or too cold. In general babies need less clothing than parents think they need, and far less than some older grandparents suggest. The following might be of guidance:

> *On a hot summer's day:* Keep the baby shaded and in a single layer of loose-fitting clothing. A baby's exposed areas (such as arms and head) can sunburn in as little as 5 minutes so a sunhat, or shade for a pram or pushchair, is essential.
>
> *On a cooler day:* Long trousers or tights and a shirt, or a babygro with an extra jumper would be appropriate.
>
> *In colder winter weather:* A baby will need three layers plus a warm hat and a blanket to go out. In the first three months it would be unwise to keep the baby out in really cold conditions for longer than half an hour or so.

In a baby sling covered up by your coat he will be getting some of your body warmth and may need fewer layers.

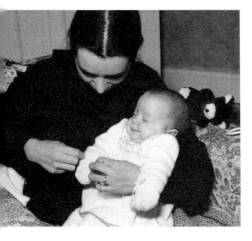

In general babies will be comfortable in the same number of layers of clothing as their parents would wear for the prevailing conditions.

In cold weather they need a warm bonnet and mittens; in hot weather they may only need a nappy and light-weight shirt.

How can I tell if he's too hot or too cold?

If a baby is too *hot* the following may be noticeable:

(1) he is sweating on his face or head;
(2) he is fidgety and irritable;
(3) he may feel hot to the touch;
(4) he may seem to be breathing faster than usual.

If he is worryingly hot then he should be undressed and covered with a light sheet, or sponged with lukewarm—not cold—water. It is best to wait until he has cooled down before giving him a drink.

If a baby is too *cold* then the following may be noticeable:

(1) he is less active;
(2) he may appear very pink, especially in the face or limbs;
(3) he will be lethargic and feed poorly;
(4) his limbs will feel obviously cold to the touch.

If placing the baby in a warm room doesn't result in an improvement *within 30 minutes* you should seek *urgent* medical attention.

Early behaviour

What can my baby do?

As we mentioned before, preterm babies, like those at term, can already see and hear. By the time your baby is ready to go home

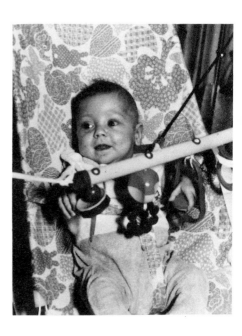

Securely supported in a sloping chair Clare can learn to play with things in front of her and see what is going on nearby.

he is probably becoming more alert and responsive to his surroundings. In these early months babies are fascinated by patterns, by contrasts of colour and light and dark, and by movement. He might look at pieces of coloured wrapping paper taped to the sides of his cot, or to a mobile made of such simple materials as coloured card or foil-covered shapes. He still sees best at close distances, so he may not notice wallpaper, nursery decorations, or the television just yet!

But you are his best 'toy' at the moment because you respond to his movements, his facial expressions, and his little 'talking' noises by gestures and vocalizations of your own. Try to give him a lot of your attention when he is awake, having conversations with him, letting him touch you, and gradually introducing him to new sights and sounds and things to hold on to. It is perfectly all right for him to sit up for short periods in a sloped or bouncing chair in order to watch what you are doing—but always make certain that he is strapped in and not left alone where he might 'propel' the chair off a high kitchen counter.

Sleeping

What should he sleep in?

From the baby's point of view it makes little difference whether he sleeps in a carrycot, a basket, a drawer, a cardboard box, or a full-sized cot, for the first few months. Certain safety precautions are necessary wherever he is put down to sleep, whether it be for the night or just a short nap:

1. He should not be left in a place where he could roll off anything such as a sofa, or out of a soft-sided basket on a table.
2. Any cot should be painted with non-toxic paint.
3. The bars of the cot should not be more than $2\frac{1}{2}$ in apart or hands and feet could be trapped. If they are widely spaced, and the baby is small, a cot bumper will keep him away from the sides, and for a particularly active baby will prevent a bruised head.
4. *Never* put a pillow in the cot or pram—a young baby doesn't need one and in rare circumstances it could obstruct his breathing.
5. The nylon 'baby nests' used for keeping a small baby warm *should not* be used for sleeping as they do not 'breathe' as bedding does and there is a chance that a baby may slip down inside.

How much sleep does he need?

Babies, just like adults, vary in the amount of sleep that they need. In the first few months the average baby sleeps 15-20 hours a day, and 3-5 hours between feeds. But some babies never seem to sleep and are none the worse for it, although the parents may well be! Many babies who have been in a neonatal unit take a while to settle into a day-night cycle since they have not been used to sleeping in the dark for many weeks. Once put to sleep in a darkened room he will gradually adjust his own rhythms.

On average babies begin to sleep through the night between 3-5 months after the date they were due, so sleeping through should not be expected too soon. Sometimes giving a last feed just before you go to sleep will reduce the number of night wakenings. But there is no evidence that putting cereal in the bottle will make him

sleep through the night, and this is not a good reason for introducing solids any earlier.

What position should he sleep in?

In the neonatal unit babies will have been used to sleeping on their
back, front, and sides. It is unlikely that he will have developed
any particular preference for one of these positions. Many babies
seem to derive most comfort from sleeping on their fronts and so
this is a good position to put him down in first. The tummy or side
position is better in case the baby brings up a bit of feed, but by
the time they are discharged from hospital most babies readily turn
their head from side to side, so that this is not a problem.

Is it better for a baby to sleep in his own room?

Where their baby sleeps is entirely up to parents and their circumstances. After missing so much of the closeness and privacy of
being together in the early weeks mothers of preterm infants often
want the baby with them day and night. They may also worry,
secretly, that if he is out of sight they may not hear him if he were
to stop breathing. Having the baby in the same room certainly
makes it easier to tend to him when he cries, and may prevent him
waking others in the house. Often there is simply no other suitable
place for him to sleep! Some parents especially enjoy having their
baby sleep in the same bed, while others balk at the idea of a wet
and wriggly bundle at such close quarters. If he does sleep in the
'family bed' it is important that he is safe; his head should not rest
on a pillow, and if he is on the outside then the sheet should be
firmly tucked around him, or a child's bedguard fastened on the
side.

There are some advantages to having the baby in another room.
Babies go through a number of different 'stages' of sleep during the
night during which they move about, or fuss and whimper, without
really waking up. An adult's sleep may be disturbed by this. Parental activities may occasionally prevent their baby from settling.
Some couples also feel self-conscious about lovemaking in the
baby's presence, but may not be able to discuss this with each
other. If the baby is really hungry he can usually be heard several
rooms away; if not a 'baby alarm' will amplify his noises from the
other room. Indeed a baby intercom can be an extra reassurance to
parents who want to be able to hear their baby's night-time noises.

Crying

Why does he cry so much?

Few things get parents down more quickly than a baby who cries a lot. Why preterm babies are reported to cry more than full-term babies when they get home is unclear, but there are probably a number of contributing factors. Firstly, the majority of preterm infants tend to go home at about 36–44 weeks' gestation, at a time when their cry has become more vigorous. Of course the baby is now mature enough to use his cry as communication with his new full-time care-givers—his parents—who have greater opportunities to respond to his individual needs than did the hospital staff.

Also home may be a lot quieter without the constant sounds of equipment and conversation in the neonatal unit, so that going home to silence will be strange. Lastly, parents often report that the crying doesn't really become a problem until the second or third week home. Again, this might suggest a maturational effect, but is also likely to be due to the fact that the family's initial euphoria on coming home has given way to the tiredness and tensions faced by all parents in adapting to the new demands placed on them.

It should be remembered that even for full-term babies crying is commonplace in the first few months. Much cuddling and patience is often needed. Two to three hours of crying a day is quite normal for some babies; in a recent study we found that 65 per cent of one month old babies were estimated by their parents to cry for two hours or more each day, and 50 per cent of the parents said that it 'got them down'. Crying seems to be most frequent in the early evening when parents are usually tired themselves and trying to do too much at once.

After a peak at 6–8 weeks in full-term infants, the frequency and duration of crying periods tends to decrease. This may not give you much consolation if you have to face 3–4 months of crying after coming home until the baby reaches the equivalent of this age. But at least it may help to realize that you are not alone, and that the crying is unlikely to be a result of the baby having new problems, of inappropriate handling, or any lack of love and caring.

But what can I do about it?

The most important thing to do is to keep things in perspective. Crying is not life-threatening and has no known complications or later consequences for the baby. But for parents who become tense and guilty about their ability to cope with what seems to them to be continual crying can eat away at their self-esteem. A baby never cries 'to get at' his parents, but he may certainly be crying for reasons that are not obvious to them, and it is often difficult to see how they can put things right.

As an initial approach you may want to work through systematically some of the 'tried and tested' methods of soothing young babies. Some babies quieten immediately to sounds: talking, singing, a continuous noise like a vacuum cleaner or washing machine, the radio or television. Because young babies often don't hear at low sound levels try a louder sound than might be normal for adult listeners.

Restraining a baby's movements, such as putting a hand on his tummy, lightly holding his arms across his chest, or wrapping him up (swaddling) in a blanket, also helps to reduce crying. Holding him upright on the shoulder is soothing in itself and also gives him a different perspective of the world. Simply carrying the baby around in a sling often quietens the most fretful of infants while still enabling a parent to get on with other activities.

An increasing number of commercial devices are advertised in magazines for parents each month, and are certainly worth considering for infants who cry inconsolably for long periods. Cassette tapes of 'womb' music, horizontal rocking cots, and vertically rocking hammocks should not replace the intimate body contact with loving parents, but they may help at times when this is not feasible.

Lastly, all parents reach a point at some time in the early months where they feel they can't stand their crying baby for another minute without exploding. When this happens it is essential to get some relief right away. Put the baby in another room and make some tea, have a drink, or run a bath. Ask a neighbour to look after him for a few hours in order to get out of the house, or take him with you to see a friend. It can be very helpful and reassuring to talk to someone in similar circumstances on a parents' 'Helpline', or on a longer term basis to join a self-help group like CRY-SIS (see Appendix 2, p. 233).

Getting out and about

When can he be taken out?

Since most babies make their first trip 'out' on the way home from the neonatal unit fresh air is obviously not catastrophic. It is probably best not to expose your baby to crowds of strangers for the first few weeks so as to reduce the risk of his acquiring colds or other infections. However, there will inevitably be shopping to do, and most mothers do not have someone on hand to look after the baby, or go out on errands for them. As long as he is dressed appropriately (see p. 164), and strangers are discouraged from looking too closely at him, there is no harm in taking him out. Because the baby has been so long in hospital there will be many friends and relations wanting to visit. If they are well the baby will certainly come to no harm, but remember that such visits can be very tiring for you!

Are pushchairs (strollers) and 'baby carriers' safe for little babies?

With an increasing number of families living in flats (apartments) and small houses the large pram (carriage) seems on the decline. Firm 'lie-back' pushchairs are not thought to be detrimental for even a newborn baby provided that he seems comfortable, is well strapped in, and does not spend more than a few hours in it. Some babies, however, will never settle peacefully unless they are lying on their tummy, or have more room to move around. Pushchairs also have the disadvantage of being more exposed to the elements, and it is usually difficult to find a satisfactory way of carrying shopping without tipping the pushchair over when it is stationary.

'Baby slings' are just gaining in popularity in Europe and America, but other cultures have always carried new babies in some sort of carrier tied onto the mother. In Scandinavian hospitals they are occasionally provided in postnatal wards to demonstrate how convenient they are for parents and soothing for the baby. It is important to use a head support in the first few months and not to put your baby in a rigid 'backpack' type carrier until he can completely hold his head up for long periods (after 6 months).

What is the safest way to take him in the car?

The only safe way to protect the baby in case of an accident is in an approved carrycot restraint system, or, in America, in a rear-

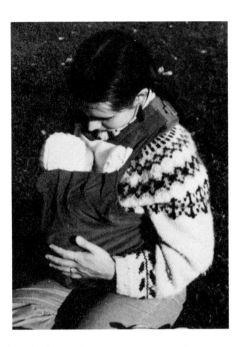

Most babies are soothed by being in a sling—and it leaves their parents' hands free.

facing infant car seat. In Britain it is often convenient to buy one of the restraint systems to which a car seat can later be attached once the infant weighs more than 9 kilos. *Never* put the baby in the front seat on an adult's lap since it is extremely dangerous, and in many countries illegal. Even on an adult's lap in the back a baby is likely to be thrown forward with the force of the adult landing on top.

Parents who say that they 'always drive slowly' forget that it is just as likely to be the other driver who does something foolish. *Never* leave a baby alone in a car; the inside temperature can change very quickly to become dangerously hot or cold.

Can he be left with someone else?

Because of the extra time separated from their baby, parents of a preterm infant are often more reluctant to leave him with anyone else. None the less all adults need some time to themselves and it may not always be practical to take the baby along. Obviously it is best to choose someone who has had experience with young babies, and you should leave a list which includes any special routines or dislikes the baby has, the place where you can be reached, and the phone number of the family doctor, paediatrician, and local hospital casualty (accident) department. Having left the baby a few times parents usually find themselves more relaxed, and less anxious and protective.

Medical matters

Parents are very aware of their preterm baby's physical character-istics and appearance having seen him often without clothing in an incubator. They may imagine that he is somehow 'abnormal' and these feelings commonly persist, even after coming home. It is difficult to accept that he will begin to look like other babies, and that transient neonatal problems will be resolved. A description of body parts and their 'unusual' features may avoid unnecessary anxieties.

The heart

Most murmurs in the newborn period are short-lived and of no importance. Occasionally they indicate the presence of a more persistent heart problem; such babies will be examined at regular follow-up appointments. Otherwise babies who have had murmurs do not need special handling or protection.

The head

The full-term baby's head is not a rigid structure and can change shape during passage through the birth canal. The bones of the preterm baby's head are even softer so that the very weight of the head can result in side-to side flattening during the weeks of lying on the firm mattress of an incubator or cot. Although the baby may have had a small, thin, 'waterpillow' in the neonatal unit to reduce this flattening, by the time he goes home his head will have become more rigid, so it is neither necessary nor advisable to use a pillow then.

There are also two noticeable 'soft spots' on the head. The first one on top (anterior fontanelle), is sometimes quite large and can be seen to move up and down when the baby breathes or sucks. It generally closes by 18 months, and often sooner. There is a smaller soft spot on the back of the head (posterior fontanelle) which can be felt occasionally.

Head growth will be routinely measured in the follow-up clinic and is an indication of both changing head shape and brain growth. It is important not to become alarmed if a well-meaning person suggests that your baby's head seems rather large as this is most often a reflection of the return to a rounder shape, rather than anything to worry about.

The eyes

By term most babies see well at a distance between 8 and 15 inches from an object, but by three months of age their attention is often drawn to bright objects further away. By this time they are usually extremely visually alert and need stimulating pictures and toys within their visual range. Some babies may have an occasional squint (seem 'cross-eyed') particularly when they are tired. This should be mentioned at the clinic so a doctor can check it. It is usually routine for babies who have been born prematurely and required oxygen to be seen by an eye specialist in the first six months since in rare instances clouding of the retina can occur (retrolental fibroplasia).

The nose

A young baby prefers to breathe through his nose rather than his mouth, so to keep his small nostrils clear of mucus he may sneeze quite often. In spite of this his breathing might still sound quite noisy, particularly during feeds. As with all newborn babies it is generally sufficient to wipe mucus from his nose since cotton wool buds may cause minor damage to the sensitive nasal lining.

The mouth

A baby's first teeth will have been forming since the eighth week of gestation and it is now recognized that dental decay is markedly reduced by providing an adequate intake of fluoride for the baby after birth. In most areas of Britain, and America, the naturally occurring fluoride levels are low, although in some communities supplements are added to the water supply. Where this is not practised, supplementation of the baby's diet with fluoride drops is recommended. These are available from local chemists, and sometimes dentists, but it is important not to exceed the recommended dose. If in doubt about local fluoride levels any dentist, as well as the local water authorities, should have the information.

From three months corrected age babies are quite adept at sucking on their fingers and this promotes a lot of salivation. Until the baby learns to swallow all this saliva, dribbling will commonly occur. These two events are not usually connected with teething, which is rare before six months. Lying on a wet sheet may cause a rash on the face but cannot always be avoided. 'Dribble' bibs should always be untied when a baby is put down to sleep.

The ears

Preterm babies have soft 'floppy' ears because there is little cartilage. They become firmer and take on a normal appearance with increasing age. As with the nose, cotton wool buds should be avoided when cleaning the ears as wax is more likely to be pushed further down the ear canal.

It is usually obvious that your baby can hear because he may be disturbed by loud noises. Occasionally a baby who has been exposed to weeks of living in a noisy, humming environment, may seem to 'tune out' sounds unless they are considerably louder, or different, from the ones he has been used to. Under normal conditions of being cared for by one person the newborn baby comes to recognize a parent's voice in the first few weeks. Therefore it is important for your baby to have every opportunity to hear the voices of his family which he will only occasionally have heard during the early weeks. The formal hearing test normally done at clinics between 6 and 9 months is an important check since hearing loss can affect later language learning.

The hair

Many babies, including those born at term, lose their hair in the first few weeks. There is no way to predict when it will start to grow again but it will eventually! Areas which have been shaved early on will be undetectable once the hair starts growing. Some babies have quite a lot of soft downy body hair (lanugo) which will disappear in the first few weeks.

The skin

Skin is important for reducing heat and fluid loss from the body, and is also an important protective barrier against infection. Whilst it is important to keep it clean it is certainly not essential to bath the baby daily. It is more important to keep the skin dry, especially around the nappy area; this will help to prevent chafing and rashes. Like any other young baby he may have rashes which come and go but any one that seems particularly persistent or uncomfortable should be seen by a doctor.

Some preterm babies may still appear to have transparent skin with rapid changes in colour (red, blue, or mottled) when they are crying or unwrapped. These fluctuations, as well as occasional blue hands and feet, do not usually mean that the baby is too hot or cold. Rather they reflect an immaturity in the control of responses to various stimuli, which will disappear over the first few months.

The chest

Babies who have had breathing difficulties in the neonatal unit will often seem to have more 'indrawing' between and below the ribs than other babies. All newborn babies have hiccups which can cause marked indrawing as well. A baby's breathing rate is affected by the level of sleep, by excitement, and by infections. It is quite normal for a baby to pause for up to 20 seconds between breaths.

Babies who have needed support on a ventilator in the newborn period seem to be more prone to develop coughs in the first year of life. Any chest infections are likely to need hospital supervision.

The abdomen

Preterm babies quite commonly have an intermittent swelling of the tummy button—an umbilical hernia—which is caused by a gap in the abdominal wall muscles. These hernias are more common in African babies. No benefit is derived from taping a coin over the tummy button; indeed it may cause skin irritation. Most close off spontaneously by the age of a year. Parents should watch out for any sudden increase in 'hardness' of the hernia associated with pain. If the swelling cannot be easily pressed back with a finger then a doctor should be consulted as a matter of urgency. Hernias which do not close spontaneously are treated surgically.

The genitalia

As mentioned in Chapter 1, the genitals of preterm babies often look very different from what parents expect. In boys the adhesions between the penis and underlying foreskin will break down normally in the first years of life. Any attempts to push back the foreskin should be avoided as it can tear this delicate area. It is not considered advisable to circumcise young preterm infants; if indicated then it must be done later as an operative procedure. The testes are not always descended at birth, and this will be checked at follow-up appointments.

By the time girls have reached the expected date of delivery their genitals usually look less protruberant. When being cleaned or changed girls should always be wiped from the front (genitals) toward the back (anal area), to avoid germs being carried up into the urinary tract.

Some common questions

Does he need any vitamin supplements?

Most of the stores of body iron and vitamins are built up in the last months of pregnancy. Babies born before 32 weeks' gestation miss out on this process, yet have a rapid rate of growth after any initial problems. They may therefore need supplementation of their normal milk diet for the first 6–12 months. Especially important during these early months are iron, vitamin A, and vitamin D which is essential for normal mineralization of bone. Some babies may also be given folic acid and vitamin E. However over-dosage with vitamins or iron can cause unwanted effects, and therefore the amount of supplementation needs to be under medical supervision. With these supplements your baby will not need any additional vitamin preparations from the clinic or chemist, so the family doctor, clinic doctor, or health visitor, must be informed about what has been prescribed from the hospital.

In Britain Vitamins A and D are available in several formulations. Iron helps to reduce anaemia that is common in preterm babies. The 'shelf life' of some of these preparations is quite short so they may need to be renewed between clinic visits, through the family doctor, or occasionally over the counter from the chemist. Like all medicines they must be kept out of reach of children.

Will he always have those scars?

Small scars at former chest drain, blood sampling, or injection sites, will become much less apparent as the child gets older. They usually disappear altogether. Should any particular scar remain unsightly it may be possible to remove it at a later date.

What immunizations should he have?

The majority of preterm infants should have the full schedule of immunizations (diphtheria, tetanus, pertussis (whooping cough), and polio) in the first year, followed by measles (plus mumps and rubella in the United States) during the second year. A few conditions in the neonatal period may be contra-indications for immunizing a preterm infant against whooping cough, for instance where a child has a history of fits, or obvious abnormalities of the brain. The majority of doctors feel that whooping cough immunization is particularly important for preterm infants because, due to past chest problems, they are more likely than other children to develop the severe respiratory complications of the disease should they contract it. In view of present increases in the number of cases of whooping cough in Britain some paediatricians are recommending that immunizations be done between six weeks and three months from birth, which may be before the baby leaves hospital.

When should I call the doctor?

Whenever you think that your baby is unwell you should seek medical advice. The first indication might be a change in his behaviour—repeatedly refusing feeds, unusual quietness or crying, drowsiness, excessive crying of a different character, or floppiness.
  It is *always* important to seek *urgent* medical advice if your baby:

   (1) has a loss of consciousness;
   (2) has a fit or convulsion (body may stiffen, eyes deviate to one side, limbs may jerk);
   (3) turns blue or very pale;

(4) develops a 'croupy' (croaking) cough, particularly in the evening;

(5) has rapid or difficult breathing (ribs stand out due to recession), or develops a snuffle;

(6) keeps on crying continuously despite comforting measures, or if his cry sounds are different from normal;

(7) remains unusually hard to wake;

(8) has an accident (e.g. falls off the bed, is scalded by tea or coffee);

(9) repeatedly vomits;

(10) has frequent diarrhoea, especially if watery (three or four stools);

(11) is unusually hot (about 37.4 °F) or cold (below 36.0 °F);

(12) has blood in stool or urine.

If, having sought medical advice, you feel your baby is getting worse, do not hesitate to tell your doctor again—even if it is the same day. If there is any difficulty in getting a doctor to see him then go to the nearest Accident and Emergency (Casualty) Department.

13

Follow-up of preterm infants

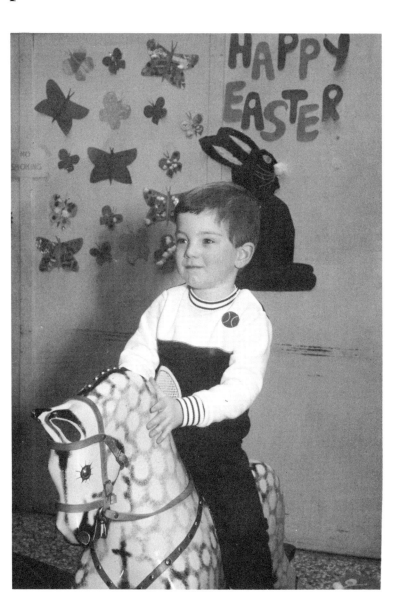

Will he be all right?

During the first days, in spite of the relief parents feel in having a live baby, many still have an overriding anxiety about the future. The attitudes of medical staff at this time may range from being unnecessarily pessimistic whenever some change occurs for the worse, to being unduly optimistic when they feel extra support and encouragement are needed. Even when provided with reassurance some parents continue to fear that their child will never outgrow his early problems, or that further difficulties relating to his early birth will emerge as he gets older. In this area of medicine, where the outcome for preterm babies is improving so rapidly, it is impossible to provide a definitive answer to the question 'what will he be like?'. The only statistical data available about the long-term effects of preterm birth relates to babies who did not receive present day intensive care.

Up until the early 1960s handicaps were common amongst the few surviving preterm babies who weighed less than 1200 g (2 lb 10½ oz) at birth. Remembering those days relatives and friends may infer that there are bound to be long-term problems for any baby born prematurely. Unfortunately child-care books and magazine articles often endorse this view.

None the less the evidence coming from ongoing studies indicates that the vast majority of preterm babies surviving today grow up without medical, physical, or intellectual problems. Advances in care have resulted in a continuing improvement in outcome for even the smallest and most immature babies, so that what was true for an earlier decade is no longer so now. A major study of babies born in the late 1960s weighing less than 1500 g (3 lb 5 oz) at birth, reported that only 6 per cent of those surviving were in special schools when followed up to school age, the rest were receiving a normal education.

The best source of information about a child's future is likely to be the paediatrician caring for him. In the early months it is not possible to give parents a guarantee of 'normality' for their baby. This is as true for a 'normal' full-term infant as it is for one who was born early. Certain events occurring in the perinatal period may increase the chance of later difficulties, but it is impossible to predict the risk of handicap for an individual baby. Only as the months pass can assurances of well-being be given with increasing confidence, or signs of problems be detected. Some of the factors that can, but do not necessarily, influence outcome include intra-cranial haemorrhage, meningitis, hydrocephalus, and severe respiratory problems.

Keeping a check on growth and development

Hospital clinic visits enable the paediatricians who were involved in the early care of a child to monitor his growth and development. Should problems be detected they can be investigated and treated. Even if your child is seen regularly at a 'well-baby' clinic or by a family doctor, hospital appointments usually provide a more specific and comprehensive check on aspects of health related to a baby's prematurity, or neonatal problems, and should be attended if at all possible. Although these visits may be frequent in the first few months after discharge from hospital, they are often only arranged once or twice a year after the first 12 months. 'Life is

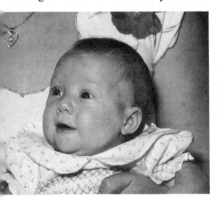
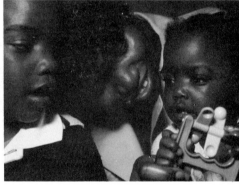
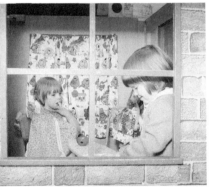
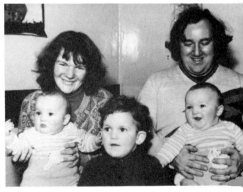

Hospital check-ups can be fun, and staff should make parents feel proud of how well their 'preterm babies' have grown and developed. Providing facilities for play during the periods of waiting makes the visit less stressful for everyone.

really great now, we don't have to go to the follow-up clinic for another six months because Joanne is doing so well.'

The exact pattern of each visit varies according to the baby's gestational age at birth, his past neonatal problems, and his current age and state of health. Paediatric departments with a particular interest in preterm babies may carry out additional checks at regular intervals, including ultrasound examinations of the baby's head. Much is also learnt from what parents say, and from observing how a baby behaves during the visit, and reacts to various aspects of the clinical examination.

A typical outpatient appointment could include the following checks:

Weight and length measurements indicate whether the baby is growing appropriately when his gestation, birthweight, neonatal problems, and family stature are taken into consideration. If a baby seems to be growing poorly then his nutritional intake is reviewed, and tests to exclude disorders which can cause growth failure instigated. These might include tests for infections, particularly of the urine, for intolerance of certain food items, and for poor absorption of dietary nutrients. The use of growth charts and the way allowance is made for the number of weeks a baby is born early, are described later.

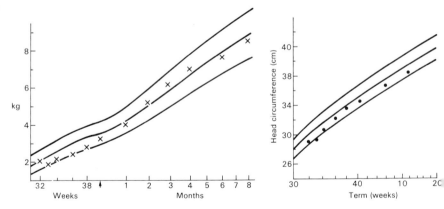

Sequential measurements of weight, length, and head circumference enable growth to be monitored. Deviation from what is regarded as normal can be readily detected and investigated. This baby's rate of weight gain increased when he went home at 39 weeks.

Measurement of a baby's head circumference with a tape measure, and plotting this on a centile chart, is a way of checking the steady increase in brain growth. Sudden increases in size, particularly if out of line with a baby's rate of gain in weight, may reflect an increase in pressure within the head. An experienced paediatrician can gain an impression of raised intracranial pressure both by feeling the tension of the fontanelle, and checking for any abnormal separation of the bones of the head. Ultrasound and CT scans can also be arranged in order to exclude the presence of hydrocephalus. With its increasing availability ultrasound scanning may be done routinely to document the changes occurring in the developing brain.

Assessment of vision may include an examination for squint, and an observation of a baby's ability to focus and follow a moving object. More formal tests of vision are used as the baby gets older, such as evaluating his ability to detect small objects at greater distances. The baby's eyes may be examined with an ophthalmoscope (fundoscopy), particularly if the baby was very preterm, in order to exclude the presence of retrolental fibroplasia.

Assessment of the cardiovascular and respiratory systems is made by examining the lips for blueness, by feeling the baby's pulses, and the heart's impulse, and by listening with a stethoscope for murmurs. The blood pressure can be checked with a routine pressure cuff and stethoscope, or by ultrasound. Any difficulty that the baby may be having with his breathing can be observed, and his chest listened to for wheezes, and other breath sounds that might suggest lung problems.

A baby's posture, muscle tone, and motor skills are examined, starting with him lying down, then pulling him to sit, and encouraging him to stand and support his body weight. This is to check the strength and co-ordination of his muscles. His ability to roll from front to back, to support his head and chest when prone, and the way he takes hold of various objects, can also be assessed. Often these observations are supplemented by his parents' comments. In this way an overview of his motor progress in relation to his age and gestation is gained. Intactness of the nervous system is also reflected by symmetry of hand grasp, Moro and tendon reflexes. These are elicited by the doctor tapping with his finger, or patellar

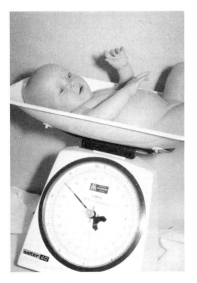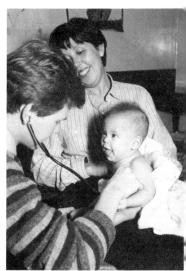

Many babies enjoy their routine check-ups.

hammer, the relevant tendons of the arm, knee, and ankle, the briskness of the jerks being noted and compared, particularly for their symmetry.

Hearing is checked by presenting a series of sounds of differing pitch and intensity to each ear. The electrical responses of the inner ear and nervous pathways may be recorded—the auditory evoked responses—using sophisticated apparatus and small electrodes placed on the scalp to pick up the brain's electrical signals. Some young babies are now being checked in an 'auditory cradle' which notes changes in body movement in response to sounds while the baby is quiet or asleep. The ear canals and drums are examined with an auroscope. Any fluid behind the drum, or infection of the ear, can be detected.

Even if your baby's hearing has been checked and found to be normal before discharge from hospital, repeated episodes of infection (otitis media), or the collection of fluid in the middle ear at some time during the first years of life, may interfere with the way sounds are conducted, and so cause a hearing deficit. If undetected and untreated, loss of hearing causes delay in speech and language development.

Routine examination is also made of the skin, abdominal organs, and genitals, and the hips are examined for stability. Special investigations may be needed to check for anaemia, and for disorders reflected in the blood chemistry. With this information the paediatrician can be certain that sufficient iron, minerals, and vitamins, are being absorbed and utilized.

Talking with parents about a baby's progress and any problems he may have is one of the most important aspects of the visit. Most parents have many questions to ask—about continuing snuffles, chestiness, a nappy rash, concerns over his rate of growth or developmental progress, and his immunizations. Pictures and diagrams may help parents understand the nature of a condition. 'The paediatrician was so nice and because he took time to explain things carefully we worried much less about our baby's problems and what might happen to him in the future.' Sometimes it is possible to relate a neonatal event to a later medical problem—for example prolonged ventilator dependence and a predisposition to chestiness; in most instances such links are less certain. Parents may get the impression that doctors are too busy in the clinic to answer their 'trivial' questions. It helps to come with a list to remind you about the queries you have. 'I felt so angry with myself when on the way home from the hospital after a visit I realized I had not been able to ask any of the questions I wanted.' If you have a problem that requires a lengthy discussion the receptionist may be able to arrange for a longer appointment at another time.

Unfortunately for some families visits to their doctor or hospital may be so unrewarding and fraught with financial, travelling, and organizational problems, that they do not find it worth attending. Cramped waiting facilities and delays at clinic, followed by only ten or so minutes with the doctor, may make repeated hospital visits seem an unnecessary claim on parents' time and patience. Paediatric outpatient departments should set an example by providing bright and cheerful surroundings, stimulating toys, an enclosed play area, a playleader to supervise activities during the inevitable wait, and to keep a watchful eye on accompanying siblings, and drinks and snacks for restless children. Limited resources mean that many hospitals can do little about their facilities and do not have sufficient staff to make the service more personal and less rushed. 'It just felt like we were being processed as we were shuttled from one doctor or expert to another. They were nice, but no one really explained anything'. Parents' groups in some areas have organized play facilities and refreshments (see the National Association for the Welfare of Children in Hospital, Appendix 2, p. 234). A hospital's League of Friends, and local charities, often donate toys and equipment.

The nature of development: correcting for prematurity

The various developing structures in the brain appear to have a well-defined timetable for maturing; the steadily changing cell and structural composition of nervous tissues within different brain regions is probably not much altered by a baby being born early. This means that a baby born three months too soon, at 28 weeks gestation, will not be sitting unsupported by himself six months or so after he was born, because by that age his brain will only have reached a stage of development similar to that of a full-term baby who is around three months of age. Although able to sit unsupported for a few moments before the age of six months, most normal full-term babies are not sitting steadily by themselves until this age or even later.

It is therefore normal to make allowance for the number of weeks a baby was born before full gestation when evaluating his development. This is so whether the kinds of behaviour being assessed are 'gross motor' skills such as sitting, crawling, and walking, or 'fine motor' skills shown in the way a young child picks up and manipulates small objects. If allowance for prematurity is not made he will inevitably seem to be 'behind' in acquiring new skills. In effect a baby is referred to as having a 'corrected', 'adjusted', or 'postmenstrual' age.

The need for this correction does not usually extend beyond two years, and may stop sooner. This is because by two years the physical growth and development of full-term babies encompasses the range and variety found in preterm babies. Although most parents realize that their prematurely born child should not be directly compared with any baby born with a similar birthdate, comparisons with other preterm infants, or with other babies growing up in the neighbourhood, are almost inevitable. Even so a baby's individuality must be recognized since his personality and temperament whether quiet, explorative, or boisterous, can also have an important influence on his development. The ease with which a child adapts to new situations can also influence the way he performs tasks presented at the clinic, and if upset by the occasion his parents' comments on his capabilities can be especially useful.

Developmental assessments

Many paediatric centres carry out developmental checks at intervals throughout the early years. One reason for doing these is to obtain information about the intellectual abilities of preterm infants and about the relationship with certain medical events such as respiratory distress, recurrent apnoeic episodes, and intraventricular haemorrhage. Long-term studies of preterm infants, around the world, have been influential in the lobbying for increased financial allocations in perinatal medicine both for research, and for care provision. Modern care reduces the chance of handicap amongst survivors, and the financial cost of handicap has been calculated to far exceed the cost of good perinatal care.

The main point of carrying out developmental assessments is to pinpoint areas in which an individual child may be doing poorly, or well, compared to his age group. Advantage can be taken of areas of increased aptitude. Similarly, in highlighting skills which are not progressing as well as might have been expected from his earlier behaviour, extra provision can be made. From the composite evaluation, the psychologist, physiotherapist (physical therapist), speech therapist, and paediatrician, are able to suggest ways in which the parents might introduce new activities, and help in the practice of others. Such involvement will encourage better progress. Opinions of other specialists may also be sought, for instance in regard to vision, hearing, orthodontic, orthopaedic, or behavioural problems.

With young babies only a few tests are used. They have been designed to measure a number of abilities in the 'mental' and 'motor' dimensions, and examine a range of skills: these include hand–eye co-ordination, babbling, imitation of sounds and gestures, physical movements, recognition and use of objects and ability to carry out instructions. The examiner will usually start with the simpler tests at a level below that expected for the baby's age, then work up to more advanced tasks, until the baby 'fails' at several of the more complicated ones. This approach enables conclusions to be reached about the spread of his abilities; for example a child may be relatively advanced in using his hands and able to put pegs into holes, or to complete a simple puzzle, but be more 'behind' in learning to talk. The information obtained also allows the tester to calculate the average age at which the child is functioning. Average age is usually expressed as a developmental quotient (DQ) on a scale in which 100 is the 'norm'. The DQ is a similar type of score to the 'intelligence quotient'—the IQ—which is calculated from the results of tests used for children of school age. However, infant tests are not as good at predicting school achievement as IQ tests carried out at later ages.

During assessment sessions a parent is usually asked to hold the baby on his or her lap because babies and young children are often quite distressed in the presence of a stranger, and by an unfamiliar setting. The tester may offer a few toys to the baby to put him at ease before introducing the test items and activities. An experienced examiner will also be able to gauge when a baby is bored or frustrated by one activity, and will then move on to something more interesting, re-introducing the original task later to see if there is greater success. Parents should try and avoid doing the task for their child, however great the temptation! However it does help if they mention similar things that their baby does at home if he seems to be failing tests that they consider to be well within his capabilities. 'I always got upset when he wouldn't do the things the psychologist wanted and threw everything he gave him on the floor. I knew he could do better at home but after the long wait it was usually hopeless.' A baby who is hungry, needs a nap, or who is just recovering from illness, is unlikely to perform at his best, and the tester may decide to re-schedule the assessment for another day.

Some paediatric departments may arrange for a child to have one or two assessments in the school years. These usually comprise standardized intelligence tests measuring verbal skills, memory, conceptual thinking, reasoning, visual-motor ability, and social intelligence. IQ measurements on a particular individual are not always definitive predictors of later success or failure. None the less any child who appears to be under-achieving in a particular area can be offered help in the form of remedial or specialized teaching sessions. Also parents can be encouraged to involve their child in dance, music, or particular sports, with a view to enhancing phys-

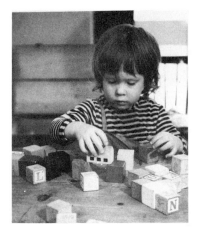
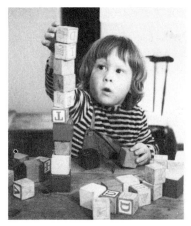
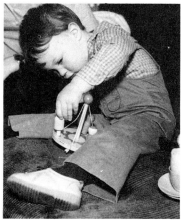
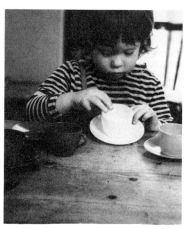

Developmental progress may be formally assessed by observing a child's hand-eye co-ordination as in building and accurate placing of objects and by giving instructions that require understanding and visual recognition as in colour sorting of cups and saucers.

ical and, indirectly, intellectual skills. These activities may help increase a child's self-confidence, and reduce the chance of later behaviour problems.

Re-admission to hospital

A few babies may need re-admission to hospital in the first year or so for planned medical procedures such as a trial with cows' milk formula, or repair of a hernia or squint. Unexpected illnesses, for example chest infections, or problems needing further investigation, such as poor growth, may require re-hospitalization. Even though parents know in advance that this may happen most are naturally anxious about a return to hospital. 'Having our prem baby admitted to hospital again so soon was very upsetting but we knew the surgery had to be done sooner or later.' They may feel guilty if their baby has again become unwell. 'I know he's only in hospital again because of a tummy-bug but it makes me feel like a hopeless mother anyway.'

Since these admissions are usually to a different ward, or another hospital, parents inevitably have to adjust to new routines and procedures, and get to know a new set of doctors and nurses. It is easy for staff on a children's ward to forget that such parents are already 'veterans' of medical technology. Parents may be talked down to even though they are quite familiar with their own baby's problems. 'I was stunned when the senior nurse told me that tube-feeding my baby was a job for the nurses since in the neonatal unit I had been told it was one of the most important things I could do for Christopher.' On the other hand nurses may also expect too much of them in this new situation. Parents with a good experience of neonatal care for their baby have a great deal of trust in medical staff and confidence in the way the baby is cared for in their absence. Others worry about what is happening to their baby even when they take a short break away from the ward. 'The nurses on the children's ward were kind but they didn't appreciate how precious Lisa was to me—after all I'd sat by her in the baby unit for nearly three months and I wasn't about to lose her now.'

Parents should always have the option of staying with their child if he goes into hospital. Overwhelming evidence suggests that hospitalization is far less traumatic if a child's parents are there with him. A few professionals, and indeed parents, feel that a young baby will not notice or be affected by the absence of his parents. This is not the case. Even a short stay in hospital can have a big impact on a baby. He is faced with many unfamiliar people, and his surroundings look, sound, and smell different. He also misses out on the familiar reassurance that parents give during cuddles, play, and feeding. If family responsibilities permit then it is beneficial to be near your child at night, as well as during the day, to comfort him if he wakes. However, as with visiting the neonatal

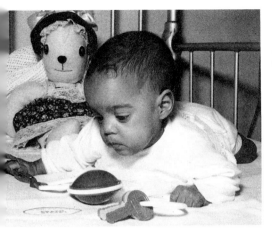

Familiar toys provide interest and security during hospital re-admissions.

unit, re-admission to hospital can pose problems in balancing the baby's needs against those of other children at home (see Chapter 10). If you cannot be with your baby all the time it is especially important that he has his favourite toys and comfort objects, and that the nurses know the way in which he likes to be fed, and how he is used to going to sleep.

In general, hospital policy has changed a great deal in recent years so that parents are considered part of the team that looks after children in hospital. Local branches of organizations concerned with the welfare of children can give advice in instances where a hospital seems unresponsive to parents' and children's needs (Appendix 2, p. 234).

In fact the majority of hospital re-admissions for preterm babies are short, and life soon returns to normal. 'Lying there in the middle of an enormous cot attached to monitors just emphasized her frailty once again, but with the support of kind and sensitive staff we got through the crisis.' 'I never thought I could bear having him in hospital again. But some of the doctors remembered Jonathan from before which made it easier, and he seemed to bounce back so quickly afterwards that a few days later he was quite his old self again.'

Types of handicap

Despite improvements in medical care some children will have handicaps as a consequence of problems associated with having

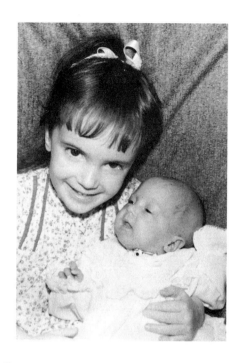

Narrowing of the trachea just below the vocal cords can follow prolonged intubation and may cause obstruction to breathing, necessitating relief by tracheostomy. The tracheostomy tube passes into the trachea below the site of obstruction enabling the baby to breathe for herself. These children can often be looked after at home until operative correction of the obstruction is carried out at a later age.

been born preterm. A handicapping condition is one which results in the inability of an individual to attain a similar level of achievement to that of his peers. The handicaps that can affect any baby whether born preterm, small for gestational age, or at full-term, can be grouped into those which involve the special senses—vision and hearing—those where motor problems predominate, those where intellectual function and behaviour are affected, and those involving other organ functions such as the lungs or heart.

Disorders involving sight, including squints and varying degrees of visual impairment, have many causes. The term 'squint' refers to a condition in which the axes of the two eyes are not parallel; this interferes with visual fixation. Squints are common in the first months, often being more pronounced and obvious when a baby is tired. They may be caused by weakness of the muscles which move the eye, by damage to the light sensitive part of the eye—the retina—or by problems which prevent the image being brought into focus. Retrolental fibroplasia causes scarring of the retina. Several factors appear to be involved in its causation; high oxygen levels in the blood reaching the retina are certainly implicated, especially if this occurs over many hours. The relative maturity of the retinal tissues and blood vessels, and their sensitivity to oxygen, may be important; occasional instances have been recorded in preterm babies where no supplemental oxygen has been given, supporting the hypothesis that the stage of maturation of the retinal tissues is of importance.

Squints that are always visible, or that persist intermittently beyond six months of age, need to be evaluated by an ophthalmologist so that appropriate medical treatment or surgery can be undertaken.

Hearing problems include any loss of a part of, or most of, the range of frequencies discernible by the normal human ear, and any problems in utilizing the information received. The former are most commonly found in association with the presence of fluid in the middle-ear, with ear infections, past exposure to high bilirubin levels, or to high levels of certain drugs, some viral infections acquired before birth, previous meningitis, and possibly with past haemorrhage in the 'inner' ear. When a paediatrician finds that a child is not hearing normally he is likely to arrange for more formal testing by an audiologist.

The development of intellectual activities and motor skills is dependent on the co-ordinated functioning of distinct areas of the brain. Intellectual impairment may become evident when there is delay in the acquisition of social awareness, when little interest is displayed in toys, or surroundings, or human contacts, and when the learning of new skills is slow. Disorders affecting parts of the brain involved in motor control may reveal their presence when children are noted to have difficulties in moving, or in control of posture; these can be due to excessive stiffness, or floppiness of trunk and limbs. Abnormalities of muscle tone interfere with the normal progression of motor development; there may be delay in being able to bring the head up and forwards when lifted from the lying position, or in balance and sitting. Crawling, standing, walking, and running, may be affected, as may the acquisition of fine motor control, necessary later on for doing up buttons, writing, and more complex integrated activities such as playing a musical instrument. Children with increased tone or stiffness are referred to as having degrees of spasticity, or spastic cerebral palsy; those in whom tone is reduced are described as hypotonic or floppy children. Some of these disorders can arise from harm done to the developing brain before birth, around the time of birth, or in later childhood.

Certain areas of the brain are more involved in the overall organization of movement than with its initiation. Damage to these areas may cause difficulties with swallowing, enunciation, postural control, or hand-eye co-ordination. Some problems do not become apparent until the child is five or six months after his expected date of delivery, although detailed neurological examinations at earlier ages may have revealed some abnormalities. Disorders associated with the development of fine motor control may not be detectable till late in the first year. Not all forms of cerebral palsy are associated with visual, hearing, or intellectual impairment. Some spontaneously resolve, with the disappearance of abnormal neurological signs by the age of seven years or so; the milder persisting forms do not prevent attendance at a normal school.

It has become increasingly appreciated over the last few years that some babies who show deviations from the normal in some aspect of development, or who display features of 'spasticity' in their first year or so, are found to be completely normal when assessed some years later. It would appear that an area of brain normally involved with one main type of function may be able to take on the functions of a damaged adjacent area, although exactly how this happens is not well understood. Only the developing brain appears capable of such great 'plasticity'. Parents should therefore be cautious about claims made for some revolutionary therapies that 'reverse brain damage'. It is usually impossible to assess the validity of these claims from the information provided by the therapists at such institutions. Careful studies have not yet demonstrated any advantages of these 'patterning' techniques over traditional stimulation and physiotherapy programmes. Since 'spontaneous' resolution of some disorders is sometimes noted, controlled large scale objective evaluation of such methods is essential.

Detection of problems in development enables appropriate treatment to be initiated so as to minimize the disability. However when the possibility of handicap is brought up the reaction of many parents is to withdraw from medical services altogether. Some justify their non-attendance on the grounds of travelling costs and dissatisfaction with cramped waiting facilities. 'I don't feel we get anywhere at the hospital visits. The doctors and medical students might learn something but I don't.' They feel let-down by the doctors, angry that handicap cannot always be prevented, or at least discovered earlier, and cheated of a rosy future for their child.

The frustrations of long waits at clinic are exacerbated by seeing other parents with their normal children, particularly if the babies were in the neonatal unit at the same time, or had experienced a more traumatic neonatal course with an apparently good outcome. 'We dread the clinic visits to the hospital . . . When you have a handicapped child, sitting there surrounded by mostly normal children is just awful.' Parents may leave home for each clinic visit hoping for a more optimistic prognosis only to come up against a matter-of-fact doctor who has nothing new to say to them.

In fact it is these parents who are most in need of a supportive, trusting, relationship with their paediatrician, and a well-organized network of support services—physiotherapists, remedial teachers, health visitors, and social workers. Communication between these experts must be good in order to avoid conflicting advice and predictions about the future. The parents themselves must always be the cornerstone of care, not only because they are with their child for much of the day, but because they know how his personality and interests can best be channelled into appropriate exercises and activities. Their love and positive involvement may eventually help to displace some of the sadness they feel, and enable them to come to terms with his limited achievements. Some parents say that the devotion evident in the way doctors and nurses cared for their baby made them aware of how precious he is whatever the degree of his handicap. In spite of the emotional cost and disruption to family life that having a handicapped child can entail, many parents find strengths within themselves which they did not realize were there.

Growth problems

Some babies, when older, may be towards the lower end of the normal range in weight and height. They may have been babies who grew poorly before birth and were small for their gestational age, or their growth may have been slow during the first few months due to the nature of their illness. Disorders arising from intolerances to certain dietary components can also cause growth failure, and these seem rather more common in babies who have been ill, or born preterm. It is perhaps hardly surprising that the immature digestive system of very preterm infants is more liable to become sensitized to foreign dietary proteins such as cows' milk, or soy protein, and such intolerances cause poor absorption of nutrients.

The rate at which babies gain weight is therefore determined by many factors. It is quite common to find preterm babies gaining weight at an accelerated rate once home, compared with when they were in hospital. Having initially fallen away from their birth weight centile they may regain or surpass it. The routine clinic checks enable doctors to pick out the baby who is not gaining weight satisfactorily. It is normal for centile lines to be crossed in an upwards or downwards direction during the first year; it is the rate at which this occurs which may identify the baby with problems.

Letting go and avoiding over-protection

Even when they know that the prospects for most preterm infants and their families are good, and observe the evidence of their own child's healthy development and intellectual progress, some parents are unable to dispel the thoughts that a disability or developmental problem is likely to show at any time. This attitude is quite understandable, particularly for those who have been through weeks of uncertainty. 'We can't help worrying about the future, even though the doctors keep telling us not to—if it was their baby they would do the same.'

Early studies on infants weighing less than 1500 g at birth suggested that their parents tended to be over-proctective, and more anxious about them, even into the school years. The authors of those original observations concluded that this 'emotional swaddling' was due to the restricted visiting and very limited opportunities for contact and care-giving that were the norm for parents in the 1960s. As policies in neonatal units were relaxed to allow unrestricted visiting, and to encourage parents to touch, handle, and even tube-feed their baby from the earliest days, it was hoped that more satisfactory relationships would result. Nowadays it seems that parents of preterm babies perceive their growing infants and toddlers as differing little in the range and variability of their behaviour from children of the same age who were born at term. 'Although we had a worrying time when she was born now she's a toddler we don't see her as being any different from her older sister at the same age.'

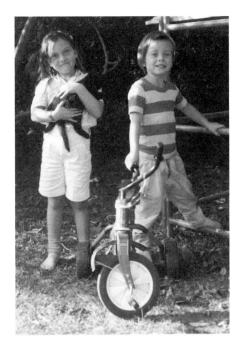

Georgina (34 weeks) at 6 years and William (31 weeks) at 4 years are just as talented as their friends who did not have the early disadvantages of preterm birth.

However, it is natural for parents to regard a child who they have almost lost as more special to them and they therefore worry more about him. But a difficult beginning to life should not keep parents from allowing their child to have the freedom to explore his environment, the chance to do things for himself and sometimes fail, the opportunities to make his own friends, and so on. He is not, in fact, more fragile or more likely to get hurt than any other young child. Having had many ups and downs in the early days can make parents fearful of taking any more chances with their child; they need to accept these feelings without letting them affect their behaviour and attitudes to their child's activities too much. Open discussions of these anxieties may help some to overcome them, with benefit to their family as a whole. 'Once he had got through the first year we worried a lot less about him, and now he has started school it's very hard to remember how small and ill he was at the beginning'.

14

If a baby dies

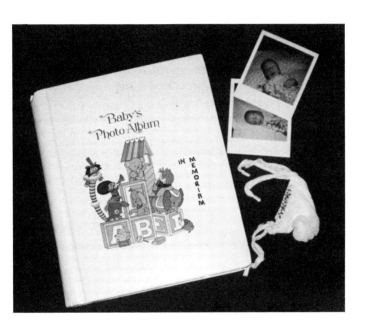

James: A perfect life

She did not want to give him up,
nursed in her womb, unpenetrably warm,
so sheltered and secure.
But when the moment of release
demanded his deliverance,
six weeks before her time,
so gently did she yield his tiny frame,
eased with such sweet reluctance
his passage to the world.
The sterile cotton, crisp and regulation white,
took over, and silence swathed him from her sight.
There was such longing for this child,
so innocent, so new,
beyond the reach of those who,
paying the penalty of love,
would never spoil him.
There was no room for joy,
but neither was there pain.
It was, after all, a telescoping of existence,
just birth and death in concertina.
His was the perfect life.

Readers may wonder why a chapter on tragedy should be included in a book concerned with the treatment, growth, and future development of preterm infants. We hope that parents will not find themselves turning to this section in their darker moments of worrying about the future of their own baby. Instead it has been written because so many parents will have already experienced one or more childbearing losses, whether they were miscarriages, stillbirths, or neonatal deaths. Their present baby may re-awaken memories and fears of previous events so that reading about the normal grief process, and of the feelings of other parents, may enable them to come to terms with what happened before. We hope it may also be of help to those who are unfortunately faced with a current tragedy, and to those with twins where one of the twins does not survive. Such parents, whilst mourning for one baby, find themselves having to prepare for the homecoming of the other.

During a pregnancy most parents at some time or other have worries about their unborn child. Early on they may be concerned with the possibility of miscarriage—particularly if this has occurred previously. Later in pregnancy a mother may be concerned if her baby appears to stop moving for a time, but once the familiar kicks and wriggles return she is reassured. Despite such worries the majority of parents are able to look forward with confidence to the birth of their baby in the knowledge that all is likely to go well.

Consequently the birth of their baby before term presents a marked contrast to their hopes and expectations. Should their baby be particularly small or sick parents may have to face the possibility of his dying. Many parents experience this 'anticipatory grief' as they fear that their baby may die. Their ability to come to accept his existence and to continue with the process of becoming involved in this new relationship may be impaired. Some may have deliberately tried to stop themselves from becoming too attached to their baby for fear that he might die, and have considered themselves prepared, emotionally, for such a possibility; even so their reactions when the loss does occur may be more extreme, and their grief more profound, than they had ever imagined.

The timing and the nature of a baby's death may cause parents to react and feel quite differently. A loss at birth, when no preparation has been possible, may seem quite catastrophic, leaving both parents in an emotional vacuum. When after a period of relative well-being a life-threatening condition develops there is time to become aware of the possible outcome. More support can be given by the parents to each other, by staff, social workers, family doctor, relatives, close friends, and clergymen. However only rarely can advance information and support fully prepare parents for their feelings and reactions at the time of the tragedy of their baby's death.

A last time together

Many parents feel a strong desire to be with their baby when he dies although they may have anxieties over what will happen, and of how they may react to such an unfamiliar situation. Others may wish to protect themselves from such an emotive event. However, afterwards, such parents often regret not having been involved in his last moments, and may want to know every detail of how he looked, and how he died. When parents have been involved in visiting and looking after their baby over several days or weeks, it may seem only natural to them that they should be doing all they can, even at the end. Many certainly achieve great peace of mind from this last act of loving someone to whom they have become emotionally attached during pregnancy and afterwards.

However not everyone is able to respond in this way. Some may find it difficult to touch, hold, or cuddle their critically ill baby, although sensitive staff can often help them achieve the necessary level of confidence to do so. When it is realized that a baby is dying it is frequently possible to remove some of the more intrusive equipment. This may be the only opportunity the parents have had of being physically close to their baby. By helping parents reach this point the almost physical ache of 'empty arms' described by some bereft parents who have never held their baby may be lessened.

If they have not already done so parents may wish to give their baby a name. This can be suggested to them, and may be an informal event; alternatively a baptism or other religious ceremony may be preferred. By giving a name parents further the process of establishing an identity for their baby so that in the future they have a 'person' to refer to and talk about.

Many hospitals encourage relatives and friends to accompany the parents in visiting their dying baby. They may be able to provide considerable support for parents in their grief. Just having other people close and joining in the bereavement can be most comforting. Sharing the new baby, even in his short life, can establish a feeling of parenthood and pride. When there are no close family or friends having a special staff member to relate to may be of considerable comfort, especially if meetings can be arranged in the weeks after the baby has died. Being able to talk to someone who has known their baby closely can provide an important outlet for the expression of their feelings afterwards.

Seeing their baby who has died

Families vary as to when their grieving begins; seeing and holding their baby are unquestionably very emotional activities and may help parents to release some of the pent-up feelings. It also provides them with opportunities of saying 'good-bye' to their baby.

When parents are asked whether they would like to see and hold their dead baby the initial feeling may be one of reluctance. Some need reassurance as to how the baby will look. After he has died a baby will be swaddled in a blanket and, although pale, will have a calm expression and closed eyes. If at all possible father and mother should be encouraged to be together at the time. If just the father is to see their baby the emotional burden of being alone, and of having to relay back details of his experience, is a heavy one. On occasions this may be the only course open to parents, but being accompanied by a friend or social worker reduces the burden. Seeing the baby in this way helps him come to accept the reality of his baby's death and enables him to provide reassurance and support for his partner.

After death all the tubes and monitor leads are removed so that for a couple seeing their baby the sight is likely to be less awesome and frightening than it may have been for them when he was alive. Their memories of him in life as possibly seeming small and frail will be modified when they see just how 'beautiful' and 'perfect' he in fact is. Sharing this last experience together quietly, uninterrupted, and for as long as they may wish, may lessen the anxieties and feelings of guilt and depression that sometimes arise later.

A few parents, despite sensitive support, feel unable to see or to hold their baby, and their wishes must be respected. Some will later appreciate a record, such as a photograph taken after their baby has died, and this can be kept in the hospital notes until such time as they request it. For them this can be a tangible reminder of the presence in their lives of another being, a true member of their family. Others may want to do or have something 'special' to remember him by. Should they want the baby dressed in cherished baby clothes, or to have a lock of his hair to keep, they should not be made to feel that these are unnatural requests.

Parents' feelings

There are some features that are common to the experience of all parents who lose a child. An initial feeling of numbness may last for a few days, during which they may behave as though nothing has happened. This is replaced, sometimes within hours, by quite overwhelming physical sensations of acute grief. These periods of profound emotional upset, which tend to come in waves lasting up to an hour or so, are often accompanied by feelings of faintness, chest pains, shortness of breath, tiredness, exhaustion, and even desperation. Although parents, and particularly the mother, may be offered tranquillizers and sedatives at this time, many professionals experienced in working with recently bereaved parents feel that the use of such drugs reduces the ability of the parent to work through the pain of the experience. Talking about and accepting the depth of feeling, and the natural consequences—tearfulness, guilt feelings, and even worthlessness—'I couldn't even keep my baby alive'—may be better than relying on drugs. Memories of this time are often fragmentary, although particular moments may be recalled with great clarity.

The waves of distress and of longing for the baby may persist for many weeks and can be precipitated by quite trivial and impersonal reminders of the loss—a child's toy, a newspaper article, television programme, or casual remark. The intensity of the feelings wanes with time as the process of mourning evolves over six to nine months. Many symptoms such as loss of appetite, sleep disturbance, irrational irritability, lack of ability to concentrate, or do necessary routine household tasks as conscientiously as before, continue through this period. Hours may be spent totally preoccupied with thoughts about the baby.

A further problem for mothers who had been hoping to establish breast-feeding, and who had therefore been using a mechanical or hand pump to express their milk, is the continued production of breast milk. As well as the psychological distress there may be physical discomfort from breast engorgement. The sensation of wanting, and of physically needing to feed the baby who is no longer there, can be one of the saddest and most upsetting aspects of their loss. Medication is sometimes needed to suppress lactation and alleviate the breast discomfort.

Anger, blame, and suppression of feelings

The anger that many parents feel initially and their assignment of blame, may be particularly hard for medical staff to cope with. The continued search for explanations as to why the baby should have died, and of how things might have turned out differently, may continue for weeks. In talking to the hospital staff the same questions may come up again and again as a manifestation of the level of preoccupation with their baby's death.

Some parents feel that the only way to deal with the crisis they are experiencing is to suppress their emotions, to try and behave quite normally, and to avoid discussing the subject if at all possible. This attitude, whilst understandable, places a great strain on their relationship and, instead of bringing them closer together in support of each other, can make them distant and unable to communicate. It is one of the roles of a friend, social worker or counsellor in this field, to help such couples bring out their hidden feelings and so come through the mourning experience. Fathers in western societies find it particularly hard to express their emotions. Not only may it be considered 'unmanly' to be seen to cry but a father, in feeling himself responsible for his family's security, may not wish to hurt or upset his partner any further. Unfortunately this reaction may be interpreted by the mother as an uncaring attitude, a sign of the father being relatively unaffected by the baby's death. Consequently she comes to feel yet more isolated in her unhappiness.

The single mother

Perhaps most vulnerable at this time is the single mother since she may feel, or even have had it suggested to her, that her baby's dying was a punishment for being born out of wedlock. Casual, sometimes well-intentional remarks can be particularly painful—'It really is for the best', 'You won't be so tied down'. Support from family, from friends, or a social worker, may help her to express her feelings, grief, and anger, which might otherwise jeopardize her future as a successful parent.

Losing a baby after a multiple birth

More complex is the situation parents face when one or more of their twins or triplets do not survive. Again, casual remarks, implying that they should be glad that they have a baby to bring home in spite of the loss of another, cause anguish. The balance between behaving joyfully towards their living infant, whilst still grieving for the one lost, is not an easy one to achieve. Setting aside certain times of the day to talk through their feelings to each other is as near as they can come to the mourning experience of other parents. Ensuring that the baby who has died retains a place within the family—perhaps by keeping his photographs in a special album—facilitates the recall of memories of him.

Older children

Parents are often uneasy about explaining the death of a baby to their other children, and may hesitate to mention it at all unless the children ask direct questions. Children need to be given the opportunity to express their feelings about the sudden disappearance of their expected brother or sister. Many of them will have been openly involved in sharing the family experience of a new baby; they may have touched or held him. The varied reactions of older children to the birth of a preterm brother or sister as discussed in Chapter 10 give some indication of how children may react to the anxiety and stress provoked by an early birth. When the brother or sister then dies, the parents are faced not only with their own emotions and reactions but with the task of trying to explain events at their children's level of understanding. The emptiness and internal conflict that parents themselves feel can unfortunately make it hard for them to provide the support that their other children need at such a time. They may be uncertain as to how much of their own emotions to reveal. If parents can bring themselves to discuss their own sadness, disbelief, and loneliness, the child may be able to bring out his own feelings and fears. Young children may be convinced that their thoughts and wishes result in actions and may therefore feel guilt that it was their wishes in not wanting the baby to come home that caused the baby to die. They may even fear that they themselves may die. Sharing their grief in fact helps to bring a family closer together and contributes to a child's ability to face later crises without necessarily suppressing all feeling or developing an emotional disturbance.

Reactions of medical staff

When a baby dies after living several days, or even weeks, feelings akin to the baby's own parents' bereavement may be experienced by nurses and doctors who have been closely involved in his care. Yet they are naturally amongst the individuals to whom parents turn for help, answers, and comfort. A sympathetic medical explanation of the events surrounding their baby's death is generally welcomed by parents.

In order to provide this bereavement support doctors and nurses feel that they have to suppress their own emotional involvement at a time when they may be feeling guilt and disappointment at the medical failure. The self-protecting defence mechanisms that are part of our subconscious may in fact distance staff from parents and result in neglect of parents' needs, or inability to recognize their signals for help. Apparently good reasons for seeing little of the parents may be proffered, particularly if parental anger is anticipated, in spite of what may have been weeks of devoted care by staff.

Some staff may be able to express their emotions to the parents or to their colleagues. However others have found the presence of an experienced counsellor at formal neonatal unit meetings to be of great value in releasing their suppressed feelings.

It should be seen as the responsibility of one or two individuals who had come to know the parents best—whether they are a nurse, doctor, or social worker—to help the parents through the initial stages of their grief. Long-term involvement is also needed. The expression of genuine feelings of distress and sympathy by staff can be of considerable comfort to parents.

Like parents, staff wonder whether there was anything that they did or omitted to do that might have made a difference. A natural reaction when parents ask questions about why things went wrong is to become defensive. Nurses and doctors have to guard against allowing professional 'tact' from preventing them giving the support that parents need. When their baby has died most parents wish to know as much as possible about 'why'; this is for their own peace of mind and, importantly, in relation to their childbearing future. Although they may be shocked and angry at what has happened, a truthful, comprehensible explanation, should be provided.

Considerable patience may be required in dealing with all the questions parents have at such a stressful time. Parents are rarely in a sufficiently calm state to remember all that is said to them. Several return visits may be needed to ensure that they have fully understood all the explanations given. It is common practice for the consultant or senior doctor to arrange these visits a few weeks after the baby's death, and then again some months later. These discussions aim to help parents to communicate with one another, and to ask any questions that they have been holding back. Providing a forum for release of pent-up emotions is another objective of such meetings. Although these follow-up sessions evoke painful memories, and many parents find it difficult to return to the hospital, they help to correct any persisting misconceptions. Social workers and counsellors experienced in working with families have an invaluable role to play in listening and giving advice over this period, particularly where parents' anger at the handling of their baby's illness makes them unable to talk over his death with the medical staff.

Friends and relations

There is an easily understood tendency for professional acquaintances, friends, and family, to behave and talk as if the baby had never existed. Many people simply do not realize that the death of a very young newborn baby is a tragedy for a family and that it usually evokes a very strong mourning response. Often the attitude is that 'You can always have another one' or 'It's better like this because the baby might well have been handicapped anyway'. These views and sentiments are sometimes expressed to parents in an effort to comfort them but they can, in reality, be quite devastating. They serve to reinforce in the parents' minds the ideas that 'no-one understands' or that they themselves must be abnormal to be so upset. Acceptance of the grieving parents' feelings and behaviour, together with sensitive discussion, especially when initiated by a close and sympathetic friend or relative, can be very reassuring. Ideally the individual should be available outside 'working hours' and in later years may share in the happier outcome of a future pregnancy.

In some areas parents have set up 'self-help' groups to provide advice and support for others in a similar situation. The isolation which comes with this kind of personal tragedy can often be lessened for some if they join such a group; there they can talk to other parents, share their own feelings, and even read the diaries of others who have come through the experience.

In some instances, however, the grief reactions amount to a severe depression preventing the individual from continuing with family commitments, work, and other activities. Professional psychiatric guidance and assistance may then be needed, and can be arranged by the paediatrician, or social worker, or through the family doctor.

Post-mortem

Soon after their baby has died parents will usually be asked if they are prepared to consent to a specialist examination of their baby (post-mortem). Although most parents realize just how important it may be to know as much as possible about why their baby died and, in particular, whether he was otherwise 'normal', some feel that their baby has 'suffered' enough and that any further interference is more than they can bear.

If given time, and a full explanation of the value of such an examination, some will come to realize the advantages for themselves and for any babies they may later have. Parents with certain strong religious convictions (e.g. Muslims) may be unable to accept the examination no matter how vital it may be for further pregnancies. Even a post-mortem examination by a specialist may fail to demonstrate a conclusive cause of a baby's dying; however it can exclude certain possibilities, including some inherited disorders which could arise in future infants of the family concerned. Screening in the early antenatal period of a future pregnancy for the identified disorder might then be possible.

Following a post-mortem the baby, dressed in shawl and bonnet, will not show any outward signs of the examination and no delay in funeral arrangements is entailed. The findings of the examination can be discussed with the paediatrician at one of the future meetings parents are offered.

Making funeral arrangements

Whether a family is religious or not, arranging a funeral, or simple ceremony with the immediate family and close friends attending, helps many parents whose preterm baby has died. When a baby dies soon after birth, or if he has been receiving 'intensive' care, parents may feel guilty that they were able to do so little for him while he was alive, and that a ceremony is something very positive that they can take part in now.

Hospitals usually offer certain options enabling either the parents to make the arrangements—with help from the hospital's administrative staff—or taking over for them completely. Not knowing what happened to their baby's body, or where or how he was buried, can add to the distress experienced later although, at the time, parents may have thought it was easier not to be involved. Participating in a ceremony, even if emotionally painful, has been found to be a helpful beginning for some parents and other family members towards accepting the death of the baby. The sadness and sympathy expressed on such an occasion is a very concrete way that friends can show concern for the parents, and demonstrate their belief that the baby matters.

Coming through bereavement

Nothing in life could be expected to prepare parents to cope with the devastating experience of losing their baby; feelings of grief are intensely personal and private. It is often the experience of witnessing the effect on their partner that leads to a fuller comprehension of the desolation of death. Memories of having all plans for the future destroyed—the loss of a potential toddler, schoolchild, and student, and of the break in family continuity—resurface during the years to come, especially on his birthday and the anniversary of his death. It may take considerable will-power to continue working at all due to the feelings of illness and loss of appetite.

But it is a widespread experience that, quite unexpectedly, laughter returns, a plan is made beyond the immediate future, and the world takes on its former variety. The bitter thoughts regarding the baby's death become replaced with the joy of looking back on a life, no matter how brief. And parents may embark on another pregnancy with all the potential for a happier outcome.

Looking to the future

One reason that parents want to know as much as possible about the reasons for their baby's preterm birth and death concerns what may happen if they have another baby. A mother may be sure that she will only feel whole and well again when she has another baby to fill the empty space that is there. Her partner may also think that this is the best thing for her. Attempting to produce a 'replacement baby' cannot mask their present grief and distress. A fuller discussion of the problems and worries associated with embarking on another pregnancy are discussed in the next chapter.

For those who cannot, or choose not to have another baby, the situation is clearly different. But there is relevance for all parents in the comment a mother made following the death of her baby after two months in special care: 'our grief and sadness are the price that we pay for life and loving our children'.

15

Another pregnancy?

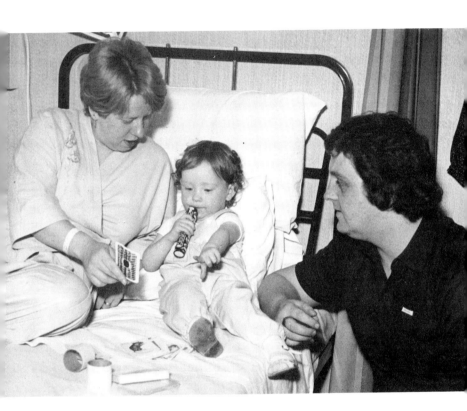

The experience of a preterm birth is not one that parents generally wish to repeat. They may worry about starting another pregnancy, about the possibility of an antenatal stay in hospital, and problems associated with the birth itself, or that their baby might need to be admitted to a neonatal unit. Their feelings about another pregnancy will obviously be influenced by what happened to them previously. Immediately after a preterm birth parents want to know how their baby is and what the future holds for him. Later, most want to know about other pregnancies and ask whether this will happen to them again.

Making a decision

If their preterm baby was very ill, or did not survive, parents often have extremely mixed feelings about another pregnancy. Many mothers describe a sense of failure after giving birth too soon— 'My body let me down', 'I feel it must have been my fault', 'I couldn't even carry her for the full length of time, perhaps I was rejecting her somehow'. Some find it difficult to face up to the possibility of another preterm birth. Other parents, following a series of miscarriages or medical problems, feel triumphant to have succeeded at all. They are usually delighted and may feel that the odds are continually improving so that they could only do better next time.

Life with a new baby is demanding, and some parents prefer not to think about having another baby until they have had a chance to enjoy their most recent one. When a preterm baby has continued to have medical problems in the months after leaving hospital his parents can feel that, in view of the concern about his health and development, they would prefer to delay having another child. Some may decide not to have any more children at all.

An 'older' couple may not want to wait very long. A woman who feels that her time is running out usually wishes to complete her family as soon as possible. Some couples prefer to have their children closely spaced and for this reason choose to embark on another pregnancy quite quickly.

Losing a baby often creates an intense longing to become pregnant once more, while at the same time it engenders great anxiety and fear about the next baby's safety and well-being. Another pregnancy should not be seen as a way of replacing a baby who has died. As was discussed in the previous chapter parents need to grieve, and begin to recover their physical and psychological equilibrium after such a tragic event, before having another baby. It is important for a family that they see the next child as a new individual with a different personality, identity, and name, from the one they lost. This can be particularly difficult should the various stages of pregnancy be experienced at the same times of the year as before, or if they hope for a child of the same sex.

Another preterm birth?

Whatever the circumstances it can take courage and optimism to begin another pregnancy. In making this decision parents, and the people who support and advise them, need as much information as possible about what happened before, and the ways in which any future childbearing could be affected. The family doctor, obstetrician, and paediatrician, need to be involved in giving parents adequate, clear descriptions and, where possible, explanations about the problems of the previous pregnancy and events that took place during the birth and the early weeks of the baby's life. Parents also need to be given the opportunity to describe how things went from their viewpoint; they may wish to ask these experts questions about the implications for future babies. Only by going over all the details in this way will they be able to achieve the peace of mind necessary before embarking on another pregnancy.

Although parents would like black and white answers to the questions they pose it is rarely possible to give these. As was discussed in Chapter 2, the reasons for any individual preterm birth are often impossible to determine exactly. With any pregnancy, 'high-risk' or otherwise, no guarantees of a good outcome and of a healthy mother and baby at the end of it all can be given in advance. However, discussions on the probability of specific problems recurring, and descriptions of the new improvements in obstetric management of 'high-risk' pregnancies, and of the advancing technology of neonatal care, can give parents the confidence to go ahead.

Only a few generalizations about the recurrence risks of preterm birth can be made. Among the disorders in which repeated preterm deliveries are likely are severe kidney disease, chronic or severe hypertension, a proven uterine abnormality, or where there has been severe damage to the cervix. With these conditions there is approximately a 50 per cent chance of another preterm birth. Other disorders, where the chances are around 30 per cent, include pregnancy-induced hypertension, apparent cervical 'incompetence', and a history of two previous preterm births of unexplained causation. Preterm birth is unlikely to recur where previously it appeared to be due to an isolated event. Examples of this are infection, physical trauma, placental abruption, or placenta praevia. There is no evidence to suggest that these events will occur again in another pregnancy.

Before becoming pregnant

Pre-conceptual planning and care is only now attracting the attention that it deserves. In no situation is it more important than in the care of mothers who are at risk of giving birth to their babies too soon. The best person with whom to discuss the detailed pros and cons of another, possibly 'high-risk' pregnancy, is the obstetrician who looked after the mother during her last pregnancy. He or she is likely to be in the best position to weigh up the past history and present circumstances, and to give a balanced medical judgement of the risks of another pregnancy, and of how long it might be best to wait.

Most family doctors are willing to write a referral letter for counselling to the obstetric unit where the mother's previous care was managed. If another hospital would be more convenient then the Royal College of Obstetricians in the United Kingdom, and similar professional bodies in other countries, should be able to supply the names of hospitals with facilities for high-risk pregnancies and intensive neonatal care. If parents have doubts about the management of their previous pregnancy and delivery, or question the competence and sympathies of the neonatal unit in which their baby was cared for, then efforts should be made to find a doctor and neonatal unit in whom they can place their trust.

Where a mother has lost one or more babies in the same hospital she may prefer to book at another hospital for her antenatal care and delivery. Parents sometimes say that they could not face walking down the same corridors again, or even seeing and talking to the same staff as before. Others, having established a positive and rewarding relationship with the doctors and nurses during the previous pregnancy and birth feel supported and encouraged by attending the same hospital, and even having their second preterm baby cared for in the same neonatal unit. However where couples have experienced a miscarriage, stillbirth, or neonatal death, it is considerate to ask if they have any preference about the hospital or consultant who might look after them during the next pregnancy. Reducing the fear and anxiety of parents who want to 'shop around', more than outweighs the inconvenience and occasional antagonism of the doctors involved.

Having chosen an obstetrician, usually with the help of their family doctor, and discussed the future pregnancy with him, a prospective mother needs to set about getting into the best physical health possible before attempting to conceive again. If a mother conceives within the first three months after having a baby there is an increased chance of a preterm birth following. Any pregnancy is a time of major emotional and physical changes for which parents need to be well prepared. It is therefore wiser to wait even longer than this before beginning again. Better health involves not smoking, not drinking alcohol, not taking any unnecessary drugs or medication, taking a reasonable amount of exercise, and eating a well-balanced diet. Checks for urinary tract or pelvic infections, and for anaemia, allow treatment to be given, and potential problems avoided.

The emotional and psychological readiness to cope with a high-risk pregnancy is much harder to evaluate than physical well-being. Sometimes there may be pressure on a wife to become pregnant again soon; she herself may not feel ready but her husband, family, or friends, may expect her to get on and have another baby quickly. The birth of one preterm baby, the trauma of separation from him, and the prospect of the same thing happening once more, often lead to ambivalence about trying to conceive again. These fears and uncertainties can provoke anxiety both before and during pregnancy, sometimes lasting up until a safe delivery is achieved.

When parents need additional advice and reassurance their family doctor or obstetrician can refer them to a social worker, psychiatrist, psychotherapist, or one of the other counsellors familiar to them from the previous pregnancy. Discussion with other parents who have been through a similar experience can endorse their decision, or cause them to pause and consider more fully.

Many parents after a preterm birth do at some stage have

another baby; however for some parents there is no next time. A few find that their relationship is not strong enough to stand the strain and their marriage breaks up. Others find that they cannot conceive again, and some just cannot face the stress and anxiety of another difficult pregnancy with the possibility of their small baby not surviving. Whether they cannot, or choose not, to have another child, most families in this situation do learn to adjust to life without children, or with fewer children than they would have chosen.

Feelings about being pregnant again

When a couple first discover that they are going to have another baby they may feel happy and excited, even euphoric. However quite soon they worry about things going wrong: 'I was so happy at first but then I started to think 'what if the baby isn't all right'; 'I held my breath and counted as each week went past'; 'I was so anxious, I worried that my worrying would affect the baby'; 'I bought one little outfit for the baby early on, then I decided it was better to wait until I knew he was going to be all right'. It seems that, at that time, mothers can feel particularly vulnerable and suffer more from the mood swings that occur in pregnancy. It is inevitable that after one preterm birth they will continue to worry that it may happen again despite the many reassurances from their medical advisers. Particularly when their previous baby was very preterm or sick, the parents' worries should be accepted as reasonable and justified in the circumstances. All parents cope better when their fears are brought out into the open and discussed with an understanding physician.

As the pregnancy progresses parents—more usually the mother—may dream about the growing baby or the previous one. Dreams fuelled by memories of the delivery room and neonatal unit may be quite frightening. Sharing dream experiences and talking over doubts and fears with their partner often brings relief, but is not always easy. Some parents keep their worries to themselves, not wishing to upset their partner, but also not wanting to put feelings into words: 'I worried about every symptom of pregnancy and whether it was normal or not, but I couldn't tell him about it until I felt better'; 'I just told my wife I was working too hard and getting over-tired; really I felt very depressed when I thought we might have to go through the same thing again'.

Most parents are cautious about telling other people of the pregnancy, and put off buying clothes or nursery equipment for the coming baby. Some relax a little when they reach the point in pregnancy when the other baby was born, and feel positive elation when this stage is left behind. This natural wariness should not be belittled by family, friends, or professionals.

Quite naturally a couple having another baby contrast the present pregnancy with the previous one. A mother may compare not only her symptoms and her own reactions but also the behaviour, particularly the movements, of her unborn baby. When she finds differences she may be comforted and feel that things will go differently. But at times of stress she may experience a flood of emotion, feeling depressed, and perhaps crying a good deal. For some mothers this happens when they go through the same medical checks and routines as before. Attending antenatal appointments and classes can be upsetting, particularly when medical staff and other mothers are unaware that the previous baby was very ill or died.

Going into labour, and the events leading up to the birth itself, can provoke great anxiety, especially when another preterm birth seems likely. However, some mothers who have faced this situation before are quite confident about going into labour and giving birth to another preterm baby. 'My first was premature, so I didn't worry so much about this one'; 'I'm glad he just seemed to slither out and that I didn't have a long and difficult birth'. Other mothers, especially those who have a long antenatal stay in hospital, are relieved that they won't have to wait any longer—'I knew she'd be small, but it seemed as though the pregnancy would last for ever'.

Parents who found the neonatal unit a frightening place before, and who did not manage to overcome their fears, will be distressed by having another baby cared for there. Others are reassured and confident because of their familiarity with the unit, its equipment, procedures, and nursing and medical staff.

Facing a high-risk pregnancy

A mother who has previously given birth to a preterm baby should consult her doctor on her first suspicion that she might have become pregnant. She may be categorized as 'high risk', depending on what is known of her present state of health and the reasons for the preterm birth.

The use of the term 'high-risk' indicates the need for a more intense medical surveillance of a pregnant mother and her baby than is usual for most pregnancies. This takes the form of frequent routine checks of blood-pressure, blood, and urine, clinical examinations, and ultrasound scanning to document fetal growth and to locate the placenta. Fetal heartrate monitoring in the third trimester may be carried out as an additional check on the baby's well-being. These assessments of the mother and her growing fetus allow appropriate advice about diet, bed-rest, or the need for hospital admission, to be discussed in good time.

Frequent and longer visits to the hospital, and an increased number of interventions, can give some couples the impression that the medical profession has almost completely taken over their lives. A mother may begin to feel that the baby she is carrying belongs rather more to the doctors than to herself and her partner. Other couples are relieved when the responsibility for their baby's welfare is shifted to the 'experts': 'We knew I would be in safe hands from the start this time'; 'With all that we and the doctors are doing to keep this baby, we feel as though things must go well'. One way for a pregnant mother to deal with her high risk status is to ensure that by asking questions and requesting explanations she is fully aware of what is happening to her body and her baby. Sometimes getting such information requires determination and persistence, particularly if your doctor believes it is better for parents not to know. Although some parents also hold this view, interviews with parents before and after the birth, and feedback from parents' self-help groups, indicate a better adjustment and recovery in those who have been actively involved in their pregnancy than in those who accepted a more passive role.

When there are several different obstetricians and midwives involved in a mother's care she is likely to receive conflicting advice and information, and therefore can become confused. In these circumstances it is more difficult to carry through a plan for the pregnancy than when there is continuity of care by one or two individuals. Communication of parents' worries and problems, and of any medical concerns, can then be maximized; this more personal relationship is associated with an improved outcome. In countries like the United Kingdom and the Netherlands, midwives often visit pregnant mothers at home. These midwives consider the development of a close and supportive relationship with their high-risk mothers to be an integral part of medical care. In some areas even high technology antenatal care can be taken to mothers at home; the use of portable fetal monitoring equipment in the home reduces the stress and resulting rise in blood pressure that could be harmful for some mothers attending hospital clinics.

Medical staff caring for high-risk mothers may unknowingly over-emphasize the 'problems'. This bias needs to be balanced by reminding parents of the many normal aspects of the pregnancy. Staff also need to recognize the increased emotional adjustments required in a high-risk pregnancy. Even when problems arise, their detection can be seen as a positive benefit for the outcome of mother and baby in contrast to what might have happened had they remained undetected. Allowing parents to listen to the fetal heart, and explaining their baby's ultrasound scan while they watch, are valuable ways in which technology can contribute positively to the well-being of the whole family.

Practical problems

Mothers who have been identified as particularly likely to give birth to a preterm baby may have their pregnancy managed intensively from an early stage. This can involve the insertion of a stitch around the cervix, and drug regimes to prevent preterm labour; some may be advised to have a considerable amount of bed-rest. They may be admitted to hospital for short stays, or to remain there for relatively long periods. Being away from home and family is unsettling in itself. For some mothers getting away from their busy home environment is the only way to ensure sufficient rest; making satisfactory arrangements for the other members of her family should be an integral part of such pregnancy care. Some mothers actually feel safer in hospital, particularly if they have had several miscarriages or previous very preterm births. 'I know they could do a Caesarean section within minutes if her heart rate got poorly'.

Even though problems may never materialize it is a good idea for a couple to draw up 'contingency plans' on the basis of the obstetrician's predicitions for the pregnancy. After an unexpected preterm birth most parents prefer to be able to make unhurried plans for the differing circumstances that may arise. Some of the possible difficulties to consider are:

1. What shall we tell our other children?
2. Who will take care of them if a hospital admission is required?
3. What should we tell employers?
4. What arrangements should be made if most of the pregnancy is to be spent resting?
5. Can household help, assistance with transport, or nursery care be obtained?

The extent of such problems will depend on diverse factors, including the age and degree of independence of other children, local availability of nursery and child care facilities, the parents' employment, and the willingness of friends, relatives, and neighbours, to help out. Long distances between home and the obstetric unit have considerable financial and logistic implications. Practical advice and support is often available from parents who have experienced similar situations. Contact may be made through self-help groups (see Appendix 2 p. 231) or locally through the family doctor, midwife, health visitor, obstetric or social work departments.

The effect on other children in the family

All children are affected to some degree by their mother's pregnancy, and any restrictions imposed by her high-risk status may further disrupt family routines and activities. In addition, an older child's memories and feelings about a sibling's early birth may influence his present reactions. Even if a child's behaviour the last time around indicated that the experience was upsetting, he may in fact remember the excitement that came with the new baby, and therefore look forward eagerly to another addition to the family. In embarking on another pregnancy parents should consider how much their children may be affected by the ramifications of a potentially complicated pregnancy, and whether there is a best time to have another baby.

Once a mother is pregnant again her other children should be told. This can be particularly difficult when parents themselves are reluctant to talk about a pregnancy where there is medical concern. However, older children especially need to know about any plans that are being made for them. Younger children may not express themselves so well, but nevertheless pick up a great deal about what is going on, and need to be given appropriate information. Advance planning allows a child to become settled at a nursery or playgroup before his mother is admitted to hospital. This is certainly preferable to sending him off to an unfamiliar situation when an urgent need arises. If he is to go to a child minder, regular—perhaps weekly—sessions may help him adjust to receiving care from someone else.

When a mother needs to go into hospital many parents are uncertain as to whether the children should visit her there, and if so how often. Short but frequent visits provide regular reassurance to a child, while avoiding prolonged periods in a boring environment where he is expected to be on his best behaviour. When visits are infrequent children may react each time with signs of distress—crying and temper tantrums—that indicate their unhappiness at the separation, and uncertainty about when their mother will come home. Parents should always be prepared for such reactions in their young children since they have too limited a sense of time to be able to anticipate the next visit. Once they are familiar with the hospital surroundings, and know where their mother is, and what she's likely to be doing, their behaviour will probably settle down. However problems of distance and transport may not allow frequent visits, and parents will need some private time together without their children. Some of the suggestions discussed in Chapter 10 may also be appropriate; talking about the coming baby, and what is happening to their mother in hospital, and making drawings for her, help a child cope better with this temporary separation. Having some new toys at the mother's bedside make the visits something special.

Despite the difficulties that sometimes arise after the birth of another baby, particularly following a stressful pregnancy or neonatal experience, most parents say that the intense and positive relationships that can eventually develop between siblings enrich family life enormously.

Coping with the temporary restrictions on normal living

Mothers who are advised to rest usually find it a great imposition, and some may feel quite angry and resentful, even though it has been explained to them that it is necessary for their baby's health.

By turning their bedroom into a living room, or moving a bed into the main room, a mother can still feel at the centre of things. This is a good time to learn and practise relaxation exercises, and the hospital physiotherapist is the best person to advise on which are most suitable. Many mothers use this opportunity to take up some new activities which do not require long periods of concentrated effort, such as rug-making or patchwork. Others continue their professional occupations quite satisfactorily from a hospital bed or home base.

Extra help at home either from family, friends, or from outside, is essential with a high-risk pregnancy. The hospital social worker may be able to find out about financial assistance for paid help. Friends and neighbours often rally round to prepare meals for the table or freezer, to take the children out, or to do the shopping, if they are aware of these needs. Mothers and mothers-in-law are often invaluable during these seemingly endless weeks or months, although occasionally the close proximity of relatives can become an added source of friction. Accepting offers of practical assistance reduces the burden on the partner and allows the couple more time to deal with the upheavals of such a pregnancy.

A mother who is normally very active may complain bitterly about the limitations imposed by having to take it easy! A woman who had expected, or needed, to work during her pregnancy may resent the financial strains and interruption to her career. Even so, most couples find that their unborn baby assumes greater importance in their lives than practically anything else. 'It is a very positive thing, helping a baby to grow well'.

Additional strains can be placed on a relationship if their doctor advises a couple to abstain from sexual intercourse. He may feel that this is advisable if there has been recurrent bleeding, or if the mother has been admitted to hospital in premature labour during this pregnancy. When parents are concerned about sexual relations during pregnancy they should discuss these frankly with their obstetrician or family doctor.

When to seek medical advice

When there have been problems with a previous pregnancy parents worry more during the next one. This is especially true when another preterm birth is possible. In these circumstances most parents are concerned that labour may start too soon, or that certain changes in their baby's behaviour might indicate that all is not well. When either parent is worried they should get in touch with their midwife or doctor to discuss the problem. Any appropriate extra checks can then be made on the baby's movements, heart-rate, or growth, which will either reassure parents and doctors that all seems well, or enable suitable intervention to be initiated. The mother's weight, urine, blood, and cervix, may also be checked to help build up a picture of how the pregnancy is progressing. It is better to make an extra visit to the doctor than to remain anxious at home.

The occurrence of any of the following problems may help a mother who has previously had a preterm baby to decide when to seek immediate medical advice:

(1) any persistent, dull, low, backache;
(2) any lower abdominal pains, cramping, or 'dragging' sensations;
(3) any bleeding from the vagina;
(4) any increase in vaginal discharge, particularly if it seems watery;
(5) any symptoms of a urinary tract infection: discomfort, or a burning sensation on urination; a sudden increase in the frequency of passing urine;
(6) any decrease in fetal movements over a period of 24 hours, after 24 weeks' gestation;
(7) any unexpected change from normality.

Coming to terms with a baby who has been 'at risk'

The emotional and medical problems of a pregnancy judged to be at risk can be too much for some parents to cope with; for others the thought of the baby they hope to have at the end of it all keeps them going. 'If this is the only way to have a baby then we are prepared to go through with it'; 'We don't really expect to get away with it, but somehow we just keep on hoping'; 'Every day that passes is a small but positive step forward for us all'.

If a mother has had a preterm baby before, even when pregnancy is well advanced it can be hard for her to invest a great deal of herself and her hopes for the future in the baby she is expecting.

Many couples are unable to acknowledge to themselves that they will have a live baby, and avoid talking about the time when the baby may be born, referring more speculatively to 'if the baby is all right'. This delay in developing feelings of affection for the baby is rather like the anticipatory grief mentioned in the previous chapter, only it is taken a step further back, before birth. Once the baby is born some elements of these negative feelings may still persist— 'I didn't fall in love with her straight away—it was as though there was a barrier between her and me and I couldn't quite get to her'; 'After all the worry it was so hard to get used to the idea that he was OK'. Having had a high-risk pregnancy it can be very difficult to believe that your new baby is fine and will not continue to be at risk in some way. A few sessions with an experienced counsellor— a psychiatrist or social worker who is familiar with the problems parents experience at this stage—may be helpful. An increasing number of perinatal centres, particularly in the United States, provide such support routinely.

It is perhaps not surprising that after a difficult or worrying pregnancy, possibly followed by an anxious birth and postnatal period, parents are not always immediately grateful for the achievements of perinatal medicine. However as they slowly adjust their lives to cope with the newest family member they gradually come to appreciate what has happened, and some view it all as something of a miracle.

'I thought I would never have another baby but when I got him home at last I realized that it had really been worth it, and that a difficult pregnancy was in fact a very small price to pay for all the happiness he has brought us'.

Epilogue

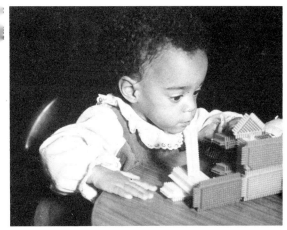

Oliver

Our three preterm babies are now well and thriving. Simone has recently had her first birthday, Oliver has started playschool, and Kim's sister is giving her plenty of encouragement.

They have every prospect of growing up as healthy, normal children, and each year thousands of babies born too early are profiting from the increasing knowledge and developments in obstetric and neonatal care.

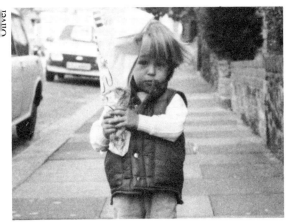

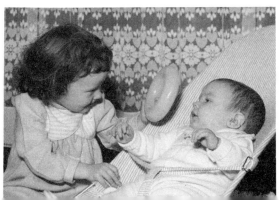

Kim with sister

Appendix 1

Practical guidance following the death of a baby (England and Wales)

Practical guidance (UK)

(1) Registration

Birth. As your baby has died after birth you will need to register the birth with the *Registrar* of Births, Deaths, and Marriages within five days. The hospital will provide the address and telephone number of the local registry.

Death. The doctor will give you a death certificate which must be taken to the *Registrar* of Births, Deaths and Marriages within five days.

The *Registrar* will give you a certificate for burial or cremation and an application form for a death grant.

(2) Burial arrangements

Whether you decide to make arrangements with a funeral director yourself, or whether you request the hospital to arrange a contract funeral on your behalf, you must take with you the certificate of burial or cremation given to you by the Registrar of Births, Deaths, and Marriages.

Making the burial arrangements yourself

You can make the arrangements by contacting a funeral director of your choice. As costs can vary considerably it is wise to enquire about the cost from more than one firm of undertakers before making the final arrangements. You must give the funeral director the Certificate of Burial or Cremation from the Registrar.

Often the hospital chaplain or your own religious adviser would be able to offer guidance over the arrangements.

Hospital burial arrangements

If preferred the hospital will usually be able to arrange your baby's burial on your behalf at no cost. The arrangements are likely to include burial in an individual coffin (or cremation if preferred) which is placed in a large grave in a part of the cemetery set aside for babies. The place will be marked by a plot number of which you can be informed later. If you wish for a service to be conducted at the graveside then you will need to arrange this with your own clergyman.

If the hospital makes the arrangements they will be able to let you know the date and time of burial so that you can attend if you wish, or arrange for your clergyman to conduct a service. If you do not wish to attend they will inform you, of the plot number afterwards if you would like that information. When you visit the cemetery it may be difficult to find the position of the plot number you are seeking if the cemetery attendant is not present. You can find this out before going by contacting the cemetery office at the Town Hall, or local District Council Officer.

Maternity grant

You are entitled to claim the maternity grant and benefit, free dental care for one year, and a death grant. You will not be entitled to claim exemption from prescription charges.

Advice

In making these decisions, it can be helpful to talk them over with different people—a social worker, paediatrician, obstetrician, chaplain, or midwife, so you should feel free to ask to see whoever you wish at any time.

Appendix 2

Information and support organizations for parents and professionals

The following list is a selection of national support groups and sources of information about child-rearing in the United Kingdom, North America, and Australia. Many of these organizations also have local branches and counsellors. A *stamped, addressed envelope* is always appreciated with your request.

General information about children and the family

United Kingdom

Health Education Council,
   78 New Oxford Street, London, WC1A 1AH. Telephone: 01 637 1881.

National Children's Bureau,
   8 Wakeley Street, London, EC1V 7QE. Telephone: 01 278 9441.

DHSS (Department of Health and Social Security),
   Alexander Fleming House, Elephant and Castle, London, SE1 6BY. Telephone: 01 407 5522.

North America

Association for Childhood Education International,
   3615 Wisconsin Ave NW, Washington, DC 20016.

Tel-Med, Inc. (Health Information by Telephone),
   National Headquarters, 22700 Cooley Drive, Colton, California 92324. Telephone: 714 825 6034.

United States Department of Health, Education and Welfare,
   300 Independence Avenue, Washington, DC 20203.

Australia

Children's Bureau of Australia,
  National Secretariat, 94 Howard Street, North Melbourne, Victoria 305.

Australian Early Childhood Assoc. Inc.,
  Knox Street, Watson, ACT 2602.

Maternity services and breast-feeding support

United Kingdom

National Childbirth Trust,
  9 Queensborough Terrace, London, W2 3TB. Telephone: 01 221 3833.

La Leche League (Great Britain),
  PO Box BM 3424, London, WC1V 6XX. Telephone: 01 404 5011.

AIMS (Association for Improvement in Maternity Services),
  c/o Beverley Beech, 21 Iver Lane, Iver, Buckinghamshire. Telephone: 0753 652781.

Caesarean Support Group of Cambridge,
  7 Green Street, Willingham, Cambridgeshire. Telephone: 0954 60630.

The Family Planning Association,
  27 Mortimer Street, London, W1. Telephone: 01 636 7866.

Foresight, Association for the Promotion of Pre-Conceptual Care,
  The Secretary, Woodhurst, Hydestile, Godalming, Surrey.

The Patients' Association,
  Room 33, 18 Charing Cross Road, London, WC2H OHR. Telephone: 01 240 0671.

North America

ICEA (International Childbirth Education Association),
  PO Box 20048, Milwaukee, Wisconsin 55420. Telephone: 612 854 8660.

La Leche League International Inc.,
  9616 Minneapolis Avenue, Franklin Park, Illinois 60131. Telephone: 312 455 7730.

C/SEC Inc. (Cesareans/Support, Education and Concern),
  22 Forest Road, Framingham, Massachusetts 01701. Telephone: 617 877 8266.

Australasia

Nursing Mothers Association of Australia,
PO Box 231 (or 5 Glendale Road), Nunawading, 3131 Australia.

La Leche League for the South Pacific,
c/o Sonya Hodder, 7 Ramahana Road, Christchurch Road, Christchurch, New Zealand. Telephone: 03 35 0908.

Parenting support

United Kingdom

CRY-SIS,
c/o Zita Thornton, 63 Putney Road, Freeziwater, Enfield, Middlesex. Telephone: 0992 716645.

MAMA—Meet a Mum Association, (National PostNatal Support),
c/o Mrs Mary Whitlock, (National Organizer), 26A Cumnor Hill, Oxford OX2 9HA.

Association for Postnatal Illness,
7 Gowan Avenue, London, SW6.

National Marriage Guidance Council,
Little Church Street, Rugby, Warwickshire CV21 3AP. Telephone: 0788 73241.

Gingerbread,
35 Wellington Street, London, WC2. Telephone: 01 240 0953.

National Council for One-parent Families,
255 Kentish Town Road, London, NW5 2LX. Telephone: 01 267 1361.

OPUS (Organization for Parents Under Stress),
Information Officer, 26 Manor Drive, Pickering, Yorkshire. Telephone: 0602 819423.

OPUS (Organization for Parents Under Stress),
Parents' Anonymous 24-hour Helpline: 01 668 4805.

The Samaritans,
St. Stephen's Church, 39 Walbrook, London, EC4. Telephone: 01 626 9000. 24-hour Helpline: 01 283 3400.

North America

Parents' Anonymous National Office,
c/o Leonard Lieber, 22330 Hawthorne Blvd, Suite 208, Torrence, California. HOTLINE 800 421 0353.

Parents Without Partners,
   7910 Woodmont Avenue, Bethesda, Maryland 20814. Telephone: 301 654 8850.

Children with Special Needs

United Kingdom

NIPPERS (National Information for Parents of Prematures—Education, Resources, and Support),
   c/o Perinatal Research Unit, St. Mary's Hospital, Praed Street, London, W2.

BLISS (Baby Life Support Systems),
   50 Sumatra Road, London, NW6.

National Association for the Welfare of Children in Hospital (NAWCH),
   Argyle House, 29–31 Euston Road, London, NW1 2SD. Telephone: 01 833 2041.

Twins Clubs Association,
   c/o J. Linney, 27 Woodham Park Road, Woodham, Weybridge, Surrey KT15 3ST.

Chest Heart and Stroke Association,
   Tavistock House North, Tavistock Square, London, WC1H 9JE. Telephone: 01 387 3012.

Aid for Children with Tracheostomies (ACT),
   c/o Susan Davies, 11 Priory Road, Market Bosworth, Nuneaton. Telephone: 0455 290718.

MENCAP (The Royal Society for Mentally Handicapped Children and Adults),
   123 Golden Lane, London, EC1Y 0RT.

National Association for Mental Health (MIND),
   22 Harley Street, London, W1N 2ED. Telephone: 01 637 0741.

Voluntary Council for Handicapped Children,
   8 Wakeley Street, London, EC1. Telephone: 01 278 9441.

The Spastics Society,
   12 Park Crescent, London, W1N 4EQ. Telephone: 01 636 5020.

National Association for Gifted Children,
   1 South Audley Street, London, W1Y 5DQ. Telephone: 01 499 1188.

North America

Parents of Premature and High Risk Infants, International Inc.,
   Maureen Lynch, Executive Director, 33 West 42nd Street, Room 1227, New York, NY 10036.

Parents of Prematures,
   c/o Houston Organization for Parent Education, Inc., 3311 Richmond, Suite 330, Houston, Texas 77098. Telephone: 713 524 3089.

Association for the Care of Children in Hospital,
   3615 Wisconsin Avenue NW, Washington DC 20016.

National Organization of Mothers of Twins Clubs Inc.,
   5402 Amberwood Lane, Rockville, Maryland 20853. Telephone: 301 460 9108.

United Cerebral Palsy Associations, Inc.,
   66 East 34th Street, New York 10016.

March of Dimes Birth Defects Foundation,
   1275 Mamaroneck Avenue, White Plains, New York 10605. Telephone: 914 428 7100.

Parents of Multiple Birth Association,
   283 7th Avenue S., Lethbridge, Alberta, Canada T15 1HJ.

National Easter Seal Society,
   2023 West Ogden Avenue, Chicago, Illinois 60612. Telephone: 312 243 8400.

World Council for Gifted and Talented Children,
   PO Box 218, Teachers' College Columbia, New York, NY 10027.

Toronto Perinatal Association,
   c/o Hospital for Sick Children, Ward 7G, 555 University Avenue, Toronto, Ontario M5G 1X5. Telephone: 416 597 1500.

Parents of Premature Infants,
   The Social Worker, Children's Hospital, S. Care Nursery, 4480 Oak Street, Vancouver, British Columbia V6H 3V4. Telephone: 604 875 2136.

Australia

The Lightweight Club,
   c/o R. Worland, 64 Surrey Road, Blackburn, Victoria, Australia 3130.

Australian Association for the Welfare of Children in Hospital,
   80 Philip Street, Parramatta, New South Wales, 2150 Australia.

Spastic Centre of NSW,
   189 Allambie Road, Allambie Heights, New South Wales, 2100 Australia.

The New South Wales Society for Crippled Children,
   Cnr. Chalmers and Bedford Streets, Sydney, NSW 2000. Telephone: 02 698 9555.

Australian Multiple Birth Association,
PO Box 151, Panania 2213, New South Wales.

Bereavement

United Kingdom

The Stillbirth and Neonatal Death Society (SANDS),
  29–31 Euston Road, London, NW1 2SD. Telephone: 01 833 2851/2.

Foundation for the Study of Infant Deaths,
  5th Floor, 4 Grosvenor Place, London, SW1 XHD. Telephone: 01 235
  1721 or 01 245 9421.

The Compassionate Friends (Support for Bereaved Parents),
  c/o Mrs Gill Hodder, 5 Lower Clifton Hill, Bristol, Avon BS6 5UE.
  Telephone: 0272 292778.

North America

The Compassionate Friends, Inc.,
  National Headquarters, PO Box 1347, Oak Brook, Illinois 60521. Telephone: 312 323 5010.

SHARE (Source of Help in Airing and Resolving Experiences),
  c/o Sister Jane Marie Lamb, St. John's Hospital, 800 East Carpenter
  Street, Springfield, Illinois 62769. Telephone: 217 544 6464, ext. 4500.

The Compassionate Friends—Winnipeg Manitoba,
  National Center, 521 Montrose Street, Winnipeg, Manitoba R3M 3M3.

Parents Experiencing Perinatal Death Association (PEPDA),
  c/o Gael Gilbert, 47 Alberta Avenue, Toronto, Ontario M6H 2R5.
  Telephone: 416 651 7422.

Canadian Foundation for the Study of Infant Death,
  181 Belsize Drive, Toronto, Ontario M4S 1L9. Telephone: 416 488 3260.

Australia

The Compassionate Friends,
  c/o Margaret and Lindsay Harmer, 10 The Outlook, Glen Wavesley,
  3150, Victoria. Telephone: 03 232 8151.

The Sudden Infant Death Association of New South Wales,
  Box 172, St. Ives, Sydney.

Medical Associations

United Kingdom

British Paediatric Association,
23 Queen Square, London, WC1N 3AZ. Telephone: 01 837 8253 or 01 837 8257.

British Association of Perinatal Paediatrics,
c/o Dr D. Harvey, Queen Charlotte's Maternity Hospital, Goldhawk Road, London, W6 OX6. Telephone: 01 748 4666.

Royal College of Obstetricians and Gynaecologists,
27 Sussex Place, London, NW1. Telephone: 01 262 5425.

Neonatal Nurses,
c/o Miss Boxall, Honorary Secretary, Special Care Baby Unit, Royal Devon and Exeter Hospital (Heavitree), Gladstone Road, Exeter EX1 2ED. Telephone: 0392 77991 ext. 325.

North America

American Pediatric Society,
PO Box 14871, St. Louis, Missouri 83178.

American College of Obstetricians and Gynecologists,
600 Maryland Avenue SW, Washington DC 20024.

Canadian Paediatric Society,
Centre Hospitalier, Universitaire de Sherbrooke, Sherbrooke, Quebec J1H 5N4.

Society of Obstetricians and Gynaecologists of Canada,
Academy of Medicine Building, 14 Prince Arthur Ave, Suite 109, Toronto, Ontario M5R 1A9.

Australia

Australian College of Paediatrics,
c/o Dr L. K. Shields, PO Box 34, Parkville, Victoria 3052.

Royal Australian College of Obstetrics and Gynaecology,
254 Albert Street, East Melbourne, Victoria 3002.

Further reading

General reading

Pregnancy

Freeman, R. K. and Pescar, S. C. (1983). *Safe delivery: protecting your baby during high risk pregnancy*. McGraw-Hill, New York.

Hales, D. and Creasy, R. K. (1982). *New hope for problem pregnancies: helping babies before they're born*. Harper and Row, New York.
(Information and guidance for high-risk mothers.)

Kitzinger, Sheila (1980). *Pregnancy and childbirth*. Michael Joseph, London.

Borg, S. and Lasker, J. (1982). *When pregnancy fails: coping with miscarriage, stillbirth and infant death*. Routledge, Kegan, and Paul, London.

Preterm care

Avery, M. E. and Litwark, G. (1983). *Born early: the story of a premature baby*. Little Brown and Co, Boston.

Bell, David (1975). *A time to be born*. William Morrow, New York.
(A physician's dramatic account of life in a neonatal intensive care unit.)

Colen, B. D. (1981). *Born at risk*. St. Martin's Press, New York.
(The day-to-day happenings in an intensive care baby unit.)

Galinsky, Ellen (1976). *Beginnings: a young mother's personal account of two premature births*. Houghton Mufflin, Boston.

Goldberg, S. and Divitto, B. A. (1983). *Born too soon: preterm birth and early development*. W. H. Freeman, San Francisco.
(Summarizes recent research findings on the development of preterm infants.)

Harrison, H. (1983). *The premature baby book*. St Martin's Press, New York.
(Comprehensive illustrated guide.)

Henig, R. and Fletcher, A. B. (1983). *Your premature baby: the complete guide to premie care during that crucial first year*. Rawson Associates, New York.

Klaus, M. H. and Kennell, J. H. (1983). *Bonding: the beginnings of parent−infant attachment*. C. V. Mosby, St. Louis.

Pfister, F. R. and Griesemer, B. (1983). *The littlest baby: a handbook for parents of premature children.* Prentice-Hall (Spectrum), New Jersey. (A question/answer format based on a description of the author's baby.
Nance, S. (1982). *Premature babies: a handbook for parents.* Arbor House New York. (By parents about their experiences.)

Breast-feeding

Llewellyn-Jones, D. (1983). *Breastfeeding—how to succeed: questions and answers for mothers.* Faber, London.
Brewster, D. P. (1979). *You can breastfeed your baby even in special situations.* Rodale Press, Philadelphia.
Messenger, M. (1982). *The breastfeeding book.* Century Publishing Company, London.

Child care

Jones, S. (1983). *Crying baby, sleepless nights.* Warner Books, New York.
Leach, P. (1983). *Babyhood* (2nd edn) Penguin, Harmondsworth. (Practical child care in relation to research findings on development in the first two years.)
Hillman, S. (1982). *The baby check-up book.* Bantam, New York. (A guide to health surveillance in the first two years.)
Bryan, E. (1983). *The nature and nurture of twins.* Baillière-Tindall, London.
Cunningham, C. and Sloper, P. (1981). *Helping your exceptional baby.* Pantheon, New York. (Practical guidance on stimulation for handicapped infants.)

Nursing, neonatal, and developmental textbooks

Auld, P. A. M. (1980). *Clinics in perinatology: neonatal intensive care.* Volume 7, No. 1. Saunders, London.
Brimblecombe, F. S. W., Richards, M. P. M., and Roberton, N. R. C. (eds.) (1978). *Separation and special care baby units.* Spastics International Medical Publications, Heinemann Medical Books, London. J. B. Lippincott, Philadelphia.
Brown, C. C. (ed.) (1981). *Infants at risk: Assessment and intervention: an update for health care professionals and parents.* Johnson and Johnson, New Jersey.
Davis, J. A., Richards, M. P. M., and Roberton, N. R. C. (1983). *Mother-child attachment in premature infants.* Croom Helm, London.

Field, T. M., Sostek, A. M., Goldberg, S., and Shuman, H. H. (1979). *Infants born at risk: behavior and development.* Spectrum, New York.

Friedman, S. L. and Sigman, M. (eds.) (1981). *Preterm birth and psychological development.* Academic Press, New York.

Hunt, M. and Blake, A. (1984). *Neonatal nursing.* Croom Helm, London.

Johnson, S. H. (1979). *High-risk parenting: nursing assessment and strategies for the family at risk.* J. B. Lippincott, Philadelphia.

Kelner, C. J. H. and Harvey, D. (1981). *The sick newborn baby.* Baillière Tindall, London.

Klaus, M. H. and Fanaroff, A. A. (1979). *Care of the high-risk neonate.* (2nd edn) Saunders, Philadelphia.

Lawrence, R. A. (1980). *Breast-feeding: a guide for the medical profession.* C. V. Mosby, St. Louis.

Marshall, R. E., Kasman, C., and Cape, L. S. (1982). *Coping with caring for sick newborns.* Saunders, Philadelphia.

Oehler, J. M. (1981). *Family-centred neonatal nursing care.* J. B. Lippincott, Philadelphia.

Prince, J. and Adams, M. E. (1978). *Minds, mothers and midwives. The psychology of childbirth.* Churchill Livingstone, London.

Roberton, N. R. C. (1981). *A manual of neonatal intensive care.* Edward Arnold, London.

Taylor, P. M. (ed.) (1980). *Parent–infant relationships.* Grune and Stratton, New York.

Conversion charts

Volume

1 cubic centimetre (cc) = 1 millilitre (ml)
5 ml ≃ 1 teaspoon
15 ml ≃ 1 tablespoon ≃ $\frac{1}{2}$ oz
30 ml ≃ 1 oz

Temperature: converting degrees centrigrade to degrees fahrenheit

	Centigrade	Fahrenheit
Freezing point of water	0	32
	35	95
	35.5	95.9
	36	96.8
	36.5	97.7
	37	98.6
	37.5	99.5
	38	100.4
	38.5	101.3
	39	102.2
	39.5	103.1
	40	104
	40.5	104.9
	41	105.8
Boiling water	100	212

Length: Conversion of centimetres to inches

Centimetres	Inches		Centimetres	Inches
25.4	10		52.1	$20\frac{1}{2}$
26.7	$10\frac{1}{2}$		53.3	21
27.9	11		54.6	$21\frac{1}{2}$
29.2	$11\frac{1}{2}$		55.9	22
30.5	12		57.2	$22\frac{1}{2}$
31.8	$12\frac{1}{2}$		58.4	23
33.0	13		59.7	$23\frac{1}{2}$
34.3	$13\frac{1}{2}$		61.0	24
35.6	14		62.2	$24\frac{1}{2}$
36.8	$14\frac{1}{2}$		63.5	25
38.1	15		64.8	$25\frac{1}{2}$
39.4	$15\frac{1}{2}$		66.1	26
40.6	16		67.4	$26\frac{1}{2}$
41.9	$16\frac{1}{2}$		68.7	27
43.2	17		69.9	$27\frac{1}{2}$
44.4	$17\frac{1}{2}$		71.2	28
45.7	18		72.5	$28\frac{1}{2}$
47.0	$18\frac{1}{2}$		73.8	29
48.3	19		75.1	$29\frac{1}{2}$
49.5	$19\frac{1}{2}$		76.4	30
50.0	20		77.6	$30\frac{1}{2}$

Weight: Converting grams into pounds and ounces (approximate), (100 grams $= 3\frac{1}{2}$ ounces)

Grams	lb	oz	Grams	lb	oz
500	1	$1\frac{1}{2}$	1900	4	3
550	1	$3\frac{1}{2}$	1950	4	$4\frac{3}{4}$
600	1	5	2000	4	$6\frac{1}{2}$
650	1	7	2050	4	$8\frac{1}{4}$
700	1	$8\frac{1}{4}$	2100	4	10
750	1	$10\frac{1}{2}$	2150	4	$11\frac{3}{4}$
800	1	12	2200	4	$13\frac{1}{2}$
850	1	14	2250	4	$15\frac{1}{4}$
900	1	$15\frac{1}{2}$	2300	5	1
950	2	$1\frac{1}{2}$	2350	5	3
1000	2	$3\frac{1}{4}$	2400	5	$4\frac{1}{2}$
1050	2	5	2450	5	$6\frac{1}{2}$
1100	2	$6\frac{3}{4}$	2500	5	$8\frac{1}{4}$
1150	2	$8\frac{1}{2}$	2550	5	10
1200	2	$10\frac{1}{2}$	2600	5	$11\frac{3}{4}$
1250	2	$12\frac{1}{4}$	2650	5	$13\frac{1}{2}$
1300	2	14	2700	5	$15\frac{1}{4}$
1350	2	$15\frac{3}{4}$	2750	6	1
1400	3	$1\frac{1}{2}$	2800	6	$2\frac{3}{4}$
1450	3	$3\frac{1}{4}$	2850	6	$4\frac{1}{2}$
1500	3	5	2900	6	$6\frac{1}{4}$
1550	3	$6\frac{3}{4}$	2950	6	8
1600	3	$8\frac{1}{2}$	3000	6	$9\frac{3}{4}$
1650	3	$10\frac{1}{4}$	3050	6	$11\frac{1}{2}$
1700	3	12	3100	6	$13\frac{1}{4}$
1750	3	$13\frac{3}{4}$	3150	6	15
1800	3	$15\frac{1}{2}$	3200	7	$0\frac{3}{4}$
1850	4	$1\frac{1}{4}$	3250	7	$2\frac{3}{4}$

Glossary

Abruptio placentae: (**accidental haemorrhage**): Separation of part of the placenta from its attachment to the wall of the uterus. May cause tenderness of the uterus, onset of uterine contractions, and bleeding. May reduce oxygen supply to fetus.

Acidosis: The situation in which there is an abnormally high level of acid in the blood due to a failure to excrete carbon dioxide through the lungs, or due to the accumulation of acid products of cell metabolism—particularly lactic acid—when the body cells are receiving insufficient oxygen.

Active management of labour: The continuous monitoring of the progress of labour, the strength and frequency of uterine contractions, and the response of the fetus as determined by the fetal heart rate pattern.

Albumin: A protein produced by the liver, present in the plasma of blood, and in the body tissues. Several drugs, and bilirubin, are carried in the plasma bound to this protein. A low albumin level may result in the formation of tissue oedema (swelling), e.g. of hands, feet, limbs, face.

Allergy: An altered state of immune responsiveness, most frequently demonstrated to dietary proteins (e.g. cows milk protein, egg, fish protein), and inhaled proteins (e.g. pollens, house dust, animal dandruff, and fur). Manifest by eczema (skin rash), asthma (recurrent wheezing attacks), hay fever, and digestive disturbance (diarrhoea and vomiting). An 'atopic' individual is one manifesting allergic symptoms.

Amino acids: The constituents of proteins—whether of vegetable or animal origin. Released during digestion and utilized in the formation of body proteins following absorption. Can be given intravenously.

Amnionitis: Inflammation due to infection of the amniotic membranes.

Amniocentesis: A prenatal diagnostic test in which a sample of the amniotic fluid surrounding the developing fetus is removed.

Amniotic fluid: The fluid (the 'waters') within the amniotic membranes surrounding and protecting the developing baby before birth.

Amniotic sac: The bag of 'waters'.

Anaemia: Too few red cells and their oxygen carrying pigment haemoglobin in the blood.

Anaesthetic: local: Medication that produces partial or complete loss of pain sensation in a given area.

　　　　general: Medication that produces total loss of consciousness and sensation.

Anomaly: Malformation of a part of the body.

Anoxia: Lack of oxygen.

Antenatal: Before birth.

Antepartum haemorrhage: Bleeding from the vagina before delivery.

Antibiotics/antimicrobials/antibacterials: Drugs used to treat bacterial infections.

Antibodies: Proteins produced by the body's immune system and directed against the foreign materials (antigens) which incite their production.

Aorta: The main blood vessel from the heart.

Apgar score: A 10 point scoring system for assessing a baby's well-being immediately after birth (0, 1, 2 for heart rate, breathing, skin colour, tone, reactions).

Apnoea: A pause in breathing: 'Apnoeic attacks'—episodes, often recurrent, in which breathing is interrupted.

Areola: The pigmented circle of skin surrounding the nipple of the breast.

Artery: Blood-vessel carrying oxygenated blood.

Aspiration:

Either - Inhalation of fluid—amniotic fluid, stomach juices, mucus, milk— into the lungs.

   or - Removal of air or fluids from a body cavity by suction.

Asphyxia: Lack of oxygen and high carbon dioxide level in the blood.

Atelectasis: Airless parts of a lung.

Attachment: The development of a close, loving relationship between parent and baby.

Bagging: The procedure of applying a mask connected to a squeezable bag over the baby's nose and mouth to achieve ventilation of the lungs.

β agonist: Drugs producing their effects by activating β type cell surface receptors—inhibit uterine muscle contractions, cause fast heart rate and tremulousness.

Bereavement: The state of having experienced the loss of a personal relationship, usually as a consequence of death.

Bicarbonate: A constituent of blood that makes it less acid.

Bilirubin: Yellow pigment in blood from red blood cells which gives a yellow colouring to the skin and plasma.

Biparietal diameter: Maximum distance between the two parietal bones of the fetal skull. (see p. 8).

Bladder: Hollow muscular organ which receives urine from the kidneys prior to its elimination from the body.

'Blood gases': Laboratory test to determine levels of oxygen and carbon dioxide gases in the blood. The analyses reflect the function of the lungs and circulation.

Arterial Oxygen Tension
   1st week: 60–100 mm Hg (8–13.3 kPa)
   Adult: 85–120 mm Hg (11.3–16 kPa)
Arterial Carbon Dioxide Tension
   1st week: 30–45 mm Hg (4.0–6 kPa)
   Adult: 20–40 mm Hg (2.7–5.3 kPa)

Blood pressure (BP): The pressure or force that the blood exerts against the walls of the arteries in the circulation.

Bradycardia: Temporary slowing of the heart rate.

Brain scan: Use of ultrasound or X-rays (CT scan) to obtain information about the brain.

Breast pump: Hand or electric device used for expressing breast milk.

Breech presentation: The position of a fetus who is bottom or feet ('footling') down rather than head down.

Bronchopulmonary dysplasia (BPD): A disorder of the lung resulting in an increased oxygen requirement and breathing difficulty which may be present for a prolonged period. Associated with a past need for mechanical ventilation.

Caesarean section: Delivery of a baby through a cut in the abdominal and uterine walls.

Candida: A yeast infection of skin and mucus membranes (mouth, digestive or genital tracts).

Carbon dioxide (CO_2): Measured as CO_2 tension (pCO_2). A gas produced in the body by cell metabolism and eliminated, via the lungs, into the atmosphere.

CAT scan: Computerized Axial Tomography. A procedure for obtaining X-ray pictures in a series of plains through the brain or other body organs, and using a computer to generate the pictures.

Catheter: Hollow plastic tube used for infusions, or to drain the bladder or other body cavities.

Centile charts: Graphical displays of the normal ranges of body measurements at differing ages.

Cephalic presentation: The position of a baby who is head down in the uterus.

Cerclage: A stitch placed round the cervix to hold it closed and reduce the chance of preterm cervical dilatation and rupture of the membranes.

Cerebrospinal fluid (CSF): Fluid produced from vessels within the brain; the fluid in the brain ventricles is in continuity with that surrounding the spinal cord. Obstruction to flow, or reduced absorption, leads to hydrocephalus.

Cervical incompetence: Early opening of the cervix, with consequent bulging of the membranes through it, resulting in repeated mid-pregnancy miscarriages, or preterm births.

Cervix: The lower entrance to the uterus (neck of the womb) which dilates during labour to allow the passage of the baby.

Chest drain: Tube passed through the chest wall to drain off air leaking from the lung (pneumothorax).

Chest X-ray: X-ray picture showing ribs, heart, and lungs; may help in distinguishing the different causes of breathing difficulty.

Chromosomes: Paired structures within each body cell that carry the genes—one of each pair is derived from the father, one from the mother. Human cells contain 23 pairs.

Chromosomal abnormality: Disorder arising from an alteration in the chromosomal make up of the cells of the individual.

Circumcision: A procedure to remove the foreskin from the penis.

Colostrum: The first milk secreted by the breast during late pregnancy and for the first days after delivery; rich in proteins and antibodies.

Complementary feed: A top-up of a breast-feed with a formula feed.

Conception: The union of the egg and sperm to create a new life.

Congenital abnormality: A structural malformation or abnormality present at birth.

Contractions: The regular shortening of the uterine muscles which cause the cervix to open and the pressure within the uterus to increase during labour, finally providing the force to push the baby through the vagina.

CPAP/CDAP: Continuous positive airway pressure/continuous distending airway pressure—delivery of a flow of air/oxygen under slightly raised pressure. Used to assist a baby's breathing and to reduce the frequency of apnoeic attacks by keeping air in the immature lung.

Crit: See haematocrit.

Cyanosis: Condition in which the skin, lips, and nails, appear bluish due to reduced level of oxygen in the blood.

Delivery: The birthing event.

Dextrose: A solution of glucose given to maintain or raise the level of sugar in the blood.

Dilatation: Opening up of the cervix.

Digestive tract: The pathway taken by food and drink, during swallowing and digestion, from the mouth to the anus via the swallowing tube (oesophagus), stomach, small bowel (duodenum, jejunum, ileum), and large bowel (colon), prior to elimination as stool (motion, faeces).

Digestive enzymes: Chemicals secreted into the digestive tract, and contained within some of the cells lining the tract, which bring about digestion of food components (sugars and carbohydrates, fats, proteins). These foods, in the form of their component parts, can then be absorbed into the bloodstream.

Donor milk: Breast-milk collected by a lactating mother and donated for feeding other babies.

Doppler ultrasound: The use of sound waves reflected off blood to measure blood-pressure and blood flow.

Drip: Delivery of fluids or blood via a needle or plastic tube into a vein or artery.

Drip breast milk: Milk that 'drips' from a breast during suckling of the other breast; can be collected and used as donor milk.

Duct: See patent ductus arteriosus.

ECG/EKG: See electrocardiogram.

ECHO: Use of ultrasound reflected from body tissues to give information about structures.

Eclampsia: A complication of pregnancy comprising high blood pressure, the passage of proteins in the urine, headaches, visual disturbances, and occasionally convulsions.

Edema: See oedema.

EEG: See electroencephalogram.

Electrocardiogram: Graphic picture of heart's electrical activity.

Electroencephalogram: Graphic display of brain electrical activity.

Electrolytes: Essential body substances that, when dissolved, are electrically charged, and give solutions able to conduct electric current (e.g. table salt—sodium chloride, potassium chloride).

Embryo: The term referring to the growing unborn baby between the second and eighth week of pregnancy.

Endotracheal tube: Plastic tube inserted through the mouth to the trachea (windpipe) to assist breathing and to allow removal of airway secretions.

Engorgement: Overdistension of the breast with milk which causes discomfort; usually due to too low a frequency of breast-feeding or milk expression.

Epidural: Regional anaesthesia used in labour and for Caesarean sections; achieved by injecting an anaesthetic drug through a fine tube sited into the epidural space of the lower spine through which the nerves relaying pain sensation pass.

Exchange transfusion: Procedure for replacing the baby's blood with adult donor blood.

Expressing breast milk: Compression of the milk-containing sacs beneath the areola to expel the milk within them—'milking the breast'.

Extended posture: Position in which the baby lies with straight arms and legs.

Extubate: Removal of the tube from the trachea.

Fetus: The unborn baby from the eighth week of gestation until birth.

Fetal 'distress': The situation arising when a fetus becomes deprived of oxygen; suggested by abnormalities in the fetal heart rate trace, and on fetal blood analysis.

Fetal heart pattern: Graphic display by fetal heart monitors; distinctive patterns are associated with fetal oxygen deprivation and other factors.

Fetal monitoring: Electronic means of displaying a record of the fetal heart rate pattern—accelerations, decelerations, and variation with the state of fetal activity.

Fetal scalp sample: Blood sample obtained by a skin prick to the fetal scalp. Used for assessing fetal pH and blood gas status in labour.

Flexion/flexed: Baby's posture in which arms and legs are held close up to the trunk.

FIO_2: Fractional inspired oxygen—in room air this is 0.21, or 21 per cent; 100 per cent oxygen is an FIO_2 of 1.0.

Fontanelle: Soft spots of a baby's head. As the bones grow together the membranes of the fontanelles diminish and disappear.

Foremilk: Breast milk which accumulates in the ducts behind the nipple and comes ahead of the main let-down reflex.

Formula feeds: Usually preparations of cows milk modified to closely resemble the chemical composition of human breast milk. Other formula feeds are vegetable based, e.g. soy formulae, or are 'elemental', comprising mixtures of amino acids, carbohydrates, fatty acids, minerals, and vitamins.

Gases: See blood gases.

Gavage: Feeding through a small tube.

Genetic counselling: Information and advice provided by experts on the detection and probability of recurrence of inherited disorders.

Genitalia: Sex organs.

Gestational age: The time (in weeks) from the last menstrual period.

Gestational assessment: Aspects of the clinical examination of a baby which are indicative of gestational age.

Glucose: A natural sugar which is a main source of energy for body cells.

Glycogen: The form in which glucose is stored in liver, fat cells, heart, and muscle.

Grief: The emotional reaction to the loss of a significant individual.

Grunting: Short rasping noises from the vocal chords heard during respiratory difficulty.

Habituation: The spontaneous diminution in response to a repeated stimulus.

Haematocrit: The volume of red blood cells expressed as a percentage of whole blood; when raised it is known as polycythaemia, when low, anaemia.

Haematuria: The presence of blood cells in the urine.

Haemoglobin: The oxygen-carrying molecule in red blood cells; too little in each red cell, or too few cells, gives a low blood haemoglobin value.

Haemolytic jaundice: Jaundice due to abnormally rapid red cell destruction.

Haemorrhage: Bleeding.

Head box: Plastic box placed over a baby's head to allow accurate control of oxygen supplementation.

Head circumference: Measurement of the maximum distance around the baby's head.

Heat shield: Clear plastic shell placed over the baby to reduce heat losses.

Heredity: Characteristics transmitted from one generation to another in genes on the chromosomes.

Hindmilk: Milk of higher fat content that follows after the let-down reflex.

Hormone: A chemical messenger which stimulates certain cell processes.

Hyaline Membrane Disease (HMD): A disorder of the lungs causing breathing difficulty due to immaturity of the production of materials which stabilize the airspaces (surfactants). Also known as respiratory distress syndrome (RDS). The lungs are unable to retain air, and under a microscope appear to contain membranes in the airspaces.

Hydrocephalus: Excessive accumulation of cerebrospinal fluid within the ventricles of the brain due to a blockage in the pathways of its circulation or absorption. May cause rapid increase in head size.

Hydrops fetalis: Excessive fluid accumulation in the fetus causing swelling.

Hyperalimentation: See intravenous nutrition.

Hyperbilirubinaemia: Raised bilirubin level (jaundice).

Hypertension: High blood pressure.

Hypocalcaemia: A lower than normal level of blood calcium.

Hypoglycaemia: Abnormally low blood glucose level.

Hypotension: Low blood pressure.

Hypothermia: Body temperature below 35.5°C.

Hypoxia: Abnormally low tissue oxygen level.

Immune system: One component of the body's defences against infections, toxins, and some potentially harmful substances.

Immunization: The induction of an altered state of immune responsiveness by deliberately exposing an individual to a material against which a future response may be desirable. The immune system is then primed to recognize and respond to the material should further exposure occur, thus preventing development of the disease, e.g. polio, diphtheria.

IMV Intermittent mandatory ventilation. See IPPV.

Incompetent cervix: A cervix which fails to remain closed during pregnancy; implicated as a possible cause of miscarriage or preterm birth.

Incubator: Large plastic box for the baby to lie in, with circulating warmed air that maintains a specified body temperature.

Induction of labour: The process of artificially starting labour by a prostaglandin pessary, by rupture of the membranes (ARM), and by intravenous infusion of oxytocin.

Infusion: Delivery of fluids or blood via a needle or plastic tube; sometimes referred to as a 'drip'.

Intracranial haemorrhage: A bleed inside the skull; this may occur on the surface of the brain, within the fluid-filled spaces (ventricles) of the brain, or into the tissue of the brain itself.

Intravenous: Into a vein.

Intravenous nutrition: Method of supplying all essential nutrients via an infusion into a vein.

Intubation: Passing a small plastic tube through the mouth or nose into the windpipe (trachea) to permit mechanical ventilation.

Isolette: See incubator.

IPPV (Intermittent positive pressure ventilation): Applying a positive pressure to a baby's airway, intermittently, to aid breathing.

IV: Intravenous.

Jaundice: The condition in which there is a yellowness of the skin and 'whites' of the eyes due to a raised level of bilirubin in the blood.

Jejunum: Part of the small intestine from which nutrients and minerals are absorbed.

Jejunal feeding: Technique for introducing milk, via a special soft tube, directly into the jejunum so as to reduce the likelihood of regurgitation or vomiting with the risk of inhalation into the lungs.

Kilogram: Unit of weight: 1 Kg = 1000 grams = 2.2 lb.

Labour: The sequence of events which results in the expulsion of the baby and other products of conception (placenta, amniotic membranes, and fluid) from the uterus.

Lactation: The secretion of breast milk; the period over which milk is secreted; the act of breast-feeding.

Lanugo: The fine hair on the body of a fetus which is sometimes visible on a baby's forehead, shoulders, and back, when born early.

Latching-on: The baby's grasping of the areola and nipple within his mouth at the start of a breast-feed.

Lecithin/sphingomyelin (L/S) ratio: Measurement of the concentrations of lecithin and sphingomyelin in the amniotic fluid, expressed as a ratio; gives an indication of fetal lung maturity.

Let-down reflex: The stimulation of contractile tissues within the breast causing a flow of milk from the nipple.

Lipids: Fats; some derived from soy bean can be given intravenously.

Liquor: Amniotic fluid.

Low birth weight (LBW): Less than 2.5 Kg.

Lumbar puncture (LP), Lumbar tap: Withdrawal of a small volume of cerebrospinal fluid (fluid which passes from the brain to the spinal cord) for analysis.

Lung liquid: Fluid secreted by the fetal lung before birth; delay in its clearance at birth is one cause of respiratory distress (transient tachypnoea of the newborn).

Lytes: Abbreviation for electrolytes.

Mask ventilation: Method of assisting an infant's breathing. A soft mask is held in place over the baby's nose and mouth, and an air/oxygen mixture flows into it from the ventilator.

Meconium: Dark greenish material that accumulates in the digestive system before birth, and usually starts being passed as bowel movements (stools) within 24 hours of birth.

Meconium aspiration: 'Inhalation' of amniotic fluid into which meconium has been passed by a fetus that has become 'stressed' prior to delivery. The sticky material irritates and partially blocks the airways causing breathing difficulties in the newborn period.

Milk bank: Location for storage of breast milk which is given to babies whose mothers do not have enough of their own.

Millilitre: A unit of volume, abbreviated by 'ml'. 5 ml = 1 teaspoon. 30 ml = 1 oz.

Minerals: Chemical elements which become incorporated into body tissues, e.g. calcium.

Miscarriage: Spontaneous ending of a pregnancy prior to 24 weeks' gestation.

Monitors: Electronic devices for displaying and recording information such as heart rate, breathing pattern, and oxygen level.

Moulding: The shape changes that occur to a baby's head as it passes down the birth canal.

Multigravida: A pregnant woman who has had one or more previous pregnancies.

Murmur: Sound of turbulent blood flow in heart or blood vessel.

Muscle tone: The resistance encountered when limbs or trunk are moved by an examiner; it arises from the resting muscle activity.

Nasogastric feeds (NG feeds): The giving of feeds via a fine soft tube passed through the nose into the stomach.

Neonate: Baby during the first four weeks of life.

Neonatology: A speciality within paediatrics devoted to the care of infants in their first weeks of life.

Necrotizing enterocolitis (NEC): Inflammation of a section of intestinal wall following damage of the lining, often associated with a period of impaired blood flow. The abdomen may be distended and blood is passed in the stools. Air penetrates the wall of the digestive tract and occasionally the gut may perforate.

Necrosis: Tissue death.

Nutrition: Term used in relation to the provision and utilization of nutrients.

Oedema: Presence of swelling due to excess fluid in tissues beneath the skin.

Oligohydramnios: Presence of a reduced volume of fluid in the amniotic sac.

Oxygen: The gas making up 21 per cent of air we breathe. Essential for normal body function.

Oxygenate: Process of providing sufficient oxygen for breathing in order to achieve saturation of the haemoglobin in blood with this gas.

Oxytocin: Hormone secreted by the pituitary gland sited at the base of the brain; induces smooth muscle contraction in the uterus and in the milk glands of the breast.

Parenteral nutrition: Supplying all essential nutrients by infusion into a vein.

Patent ductus arteriosus (PDA): The state of the blood vessel between the pulmonary artery and aorta when it remains open, after it should have closed.

PEEP: (Positive End Expiratory Pressure); positive pressure applied during expiration which helps keep the lungs from collapsing during mechanical ventilation.

Perinatal: The period from 28 weeks' gestation to the end of the first week of life.

Periodic breathing: Pattern of breathing characterized by pauses of up to 10 seconds.

Persistent fetal circulation: Persistence of the high level of muscular tone in the blood vessels of the lung which is normally present before birth. Causes diminished blood flow to the lungs and is relieved by giving oxygen, and sometimes drugs, to dilate the constricted vessels.

pH: Denotes the acidity (low value) or alkalinity (raised value) of the blood. A value close to 7.4 is normal for arterial blood.

Phototherapy: The use of light to photodegrade bilirubin in the skin and reduce the plasma bilirubin level.

Physiotherapy: For the chest, procedures are used which provide vibrations to the chest wall to help loosen lung secretions, followed by suctioning to remove the mucus from the airway. For the limbs and trunk, manipulations and exercises are given to improve muscle tone, co-ordination and posture.

Placenta: Organ comprising maternal and fetal tissues through which nutrients and oxygen pass to the fetus, and waste products from the fetus pass to the mother via the umbilical cord.

Placenta praevia: Describes the position of a placenta which is close to or overrides the outlet (cervical canal) for the uterus.

Plasma: The liquid component of blood in which the blood cells are suspended.

Pneumothorax: Presence of air between the lung and chest wall following an air-leak from a lung.

Pneumonia: Inflammation of lung tissue due to infection, or chemical irritation following aspiration.

PO: 'per os'—by mouth.

PO$_2$ or PaO$_2$: Partial pressure of oxygen in blood—provides an indication of the amount of oxygen available to the tissues.

Polycythaemia: Raised number of red cells in the blood—can make the blood very viscous.

Polyhydramnios: Excessive volume of amniotic fluid.

Posset: Small regurgitation of feed; 'spitting up'.

Postmaturity: Gestation beyond 42 weeks.

Postnatal: Occurring following birth.

Pre-eclamptic toxaemia: First stage of pregnancy toxaemia characterized by raised blood pressure, limb swelling, and presence of albumin in the urine.

Preemie: See preterm baby.

Premature baby: See preterm baby.

Presentation: Describes position of baby in relation to the outlet of the uterus (cervix).

Preterm baby: Baby born before completion of 37 weeks' gestation.

Primigravida: A woman in her first pregnancy.

Prolapsed cord: Situation following dilatation of the cervix in which the umbilical cord passes through the cervix in front of the baby—can result in cord compression and reduced amount of oxygen reaching the fetus.

Prone: The position of a baby when lying on his tummy.

Prostaglandins: Naturally occurring compounds which cause changes in smooth muscle contractility; promote uterine muscle contraction in labour, and lung blood vessel relaxation after birth.

Pulmonary oedema: Excess of water in the lung tissues—often associated with heart failure as may accompany a patent ductus arteriosus.

Rapid eye movement sleep (REM): Phase of sleep associated with reduced body muscle tone, reduced stability of the chest wall, and apnoeic attacks, especially in preterm babies.

Regurgitation: Bringing up a small amount of swallowed feed.

Relactation: Process of re-establishing breast-feeding after a period of not doing so.

Retics: Immature red blood cells (reticulocytes); found in increased numbers when anaemia follows blood loss or increased red cell destruction.

Retina: Back of eye where blood-vessels supplying the light-sensitive cells are located.

Retrolental fibroplasia (RLF): Damage to the light-sensitive retina of the eye. Causally related to amount of oxygen in blood reaching the retina, although very immature infants seem at greatest risk. Mild forms of damage are reversible; severe damage can result in blindness.

Rooming-in: The time when a mother resides in hospital and gradually takes over the full care of her baby before discharge home.

Scalp clip: Method of obtaining a record of the fetal heart rate by attaching a wire with a clip to the fetal scalp before delivery.

Sepsis: Bacterial infection.

Shake test: Performed on an amniotic fluid sample, or on stomach fluid obtained after delivery, to give an indication of lung maturity. The presence of surface active materials results in bubble stability, and is evidence of lung maturation; in their absence, bubbles collapse.

Small for gestational age (SGA): The category of infants whose birth weights are less than those of 90 per cent of babies of the same gestational age.

Squint: Condition in which the axes of the eyes are intermittently or continuously not parallel when focussed on distant objects.

Steroids: A large group of chemically related compounds of diverse origin and function. Those related to cortisol from the adrenal gland can induce maturation of the preterm fetal lung.

Stillbirth: Delivery of a dead baby after the 28th week of gestation.

Strabismus: See squint.

Suctioning: Removal of mucus from nose, throat, or airway, using a fine plastic tube connected to a negative pressure.

Supine: The position of a baby when lying on his back.

Supplementary feed: Tube or bottle-feed given after a breast-feed.

Surfactants: Compounds which line the air spaces of the lungs, reducing surface tension and thereby preventing lung collapse on breathing out.

Tachycardia: Rapid heart rate.

Tachypnoea: Rapid breathing rate.

Temperature probe: Device for recording temperature from skin surface (abdomen) or body cavity, e.g. rectum.

Term baby: Infant of between 37 and 42 weeks' gestation.

Thrush: Common name for a yeast infection (candida albicans) which can involve skin, mouth, and digestive tract; has the appearance of white patches on the surface of the mouth and tongue.

Top-up: Transfusion of blood to raise the haemoglobin level.

Toxaemia: Disorder of pregnancy comprising tissue swelling, raised blood-pressure, and presence of protein in the urine. Can be associated with impaired placental function and poor fetal growth.

Transcutaneous oxygen monitoring (T^cO_2): Device for measuring oxygen in blood passing beneath the skin surface.

Transient tachypnoea of the newborn: *see* lung liquid.

Transfusion: Infusion of blood from a donor to a recipient to raise the haemoglobin level.

Transverse lie: Position in which the fetus is lying at right angles to the outlet from the uterus.

Trimester: A period of three months; pregnancy can be divided into three trimesters.

Twins: Simultaneous development of two babies in the uterus; occurs either as a result of a single fertilized ovum dividing to produce two identical individuals (monozygotic) or as a result of the development of two independently fertilized ova to give non-identical twins (dizygotic).

Ultrasound imaging: The visual display of high frequency sound waves reflected from tissues of differing density to produce images of body organs and structures.

Umbilical catheter: Plastic tube inserted through one of the two umbilical arteries for taking blood samples for analysis of blood gas state and pH status. Some contain a device for monitoring the level of oxygen in the blood flowing past the tip.

Umbilical cord: Structure through which fetal blood flows to and from the placenta to pick up oxygen and nutrients, and to carry away waste products. Enters the baby at the navel.

Umbilicus: The navel.

Umbilical hernia: Swelling consisting of a protrusion of abdominal contents through a defect in the abdominal wall adjacent to the navel. Many of these defects close spontaneously.

Uterus: Womb; the hollow muscular organ in which the fertilized ovum implants and grows during pregnancy.

Vein: Blood vessel that carries blood from the tissues to the heart.

Ventilation: Mechanical provision of cyclical inflation of a baby's lungs to achieve normal levels of oxygen and carbon dioxide in the baby's blood.

Ventricle: Chamber—in the heart and in the brain.

Vernix: Protective, white, greasy material, covering the skin at birth, produced by glands in the skin of the developing fetus. Reduces skin colonization by bacteria after birth.

Vertex: Position in which the head of the fetus overlies the outlet from the uterus. The normal presentation at term.

Viability: Notion of the ability to survive outside the uterus.

Vital signs: Observations of temperature, blood pressure, heart and respiratory rates.

'Went off': Term used to describe episode during which a baby needed extra breathing support or resuscitation.

Wet lung: See lung liquid.

White blood count: Number of white cells (leucocytes) in the blood—used as an indicator of the presence of infection; when immature forms (bands) are present in a higher than normal proportion, infection is a possible cause.

Index